Synthesis Lectures on Data, Semantics, and Knowledge

Series Editors

Ying Ding, The University of Texas at Austin, Austin, USA

Paul Groth, AMSTERDAM, Noord-Holland, The Netherlands

This series focuses on the pivotal role that data on the web and the emergent technologies that surround it play both in the evolution of the World Wide Web as well as applications in domains requiring data integration and semantic analysis. The large-scale availability of both structured and unstructured data on the Web has enabled radically new technologies to develop. It has impacted developments in a variety of areas including machine learning, deep learning, semantic search, and natural language processing. Knowledge and semantics are a critical foundation for the sharing, utilization, and organization of this data. The series aims both to provide pathways into the field of research and an understanding of the principles underlying these technologies for an audience of scientists, engineers, and practitioners.

Guo-Qiang Zhang · Rashmie Abeysinghe ·
Licong Cui

Formal Methods
for the Analysis
of Biomedical Ontologies

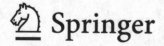 Springer

Guo-Qiang Zhang
The University of Texas Health Science Center
at Houston
Houston, TX, USA

Rashmie Abeysinghe
The University of Texas Health Science Center
at Houston
Houston, TX, USA

Licong Cui
The University of Texas Health Science Center
at Houston
Houston, TX, USA

ISSN 2691-2023   ISSN 2691-2031   (electronic)
Synthesis Lectures on Data, Semantics, and Knowledge
ISBN 978-3-031-12133-3   ISBN 978-3-031-12131-9   (eBook)
https://doi.org/10.1007/978-3-031-12131-9

This Springer imprint is published by the registered company Springer Nature Switzerland AG
The registered company address is: Gewerbestrasse 11, 6330 Cham, Switzerland

Preface

Motivation. Ontologies in general, biomedical ontologies in particular, cover a vast range of topics from philosophical to practical and from principles to applications. This book introduces an emerging area that uses formal methods, based on mathematics and logic, for the analysis and enhancement of biomedical ontologies. It takes a pragmatic approach aimed at producing actionable insights for achieving high-qualify codified biomedical knowledge in the most active and impactful areas where ontologies make a direct real-world difference.

Traditionally, Formal Methods refer to a branch of software engineering in which computer programs, protocols, and software systems are modeled, specified, and analyzed with aspired mathematical rigor to ensure that programming artifacts have desired properties. Formal methods is a term designed to distinguish it from "informal," and hence imprecise, methods. Being "formal" entails that programming artifacts, their properties, and the verification of such properties are all treated using mathematical approaches (existing or newly invented) covering both syntactic and semantic aspects. Predominantly used in the analysis and design of computer software and hardware, formal methods are particularly good at finding unexpected problems that may arise in complex systems and ensuring their safety upstream in the design phase, thus minimizing potentially catastrophic consequences downstream.

The basic thesis of this book is biomedical ontologies, similar to programming artifacts, can benefit from a similar approach using formal methods with which to find unexpected "bugs" and content materials. As the evolution of biomedical ontologies almost inevitably involves manual work, formal methods are a particularly useful tool for ontological engineering and practice. The defining characteristics of formal methods require us to rigorously formulate, analyze, and mathematically prove the correctness of algorithms for ontological analysis. This requirement also serves as a motivation for the topics, style, and content to be covered in the book.

Selection of topics. The book is a self-contained synthesis of over 30 publications by the authors on analysis (including auditing, curation, and enhancement) of biomedical ontologies revolving around a novel formal method called "formal concept analysis." Each chapter captures several related publications on a coherent sub-theme, from simple to more complex. The book is not meant to be a comprehensive review of the subject matter, nor does it strive to be unbiased in its selection of topics.

Content overview. Chapter 2 serves as an introduction to simple but formalized strategies for discovering undesired and incoherent patterns in ontologies. Chapter 3 covers the application of formal concept analysis as a formal method for semantic completeness. Chapter 4 turns formal concept analysis, a classical approach used in the mathematical treatment of orders and lattices, into an ontological engineering principle, focusing on the structural property of ontologies with respect to its conformation to lattice or not (non-lattice). Exhaustive lattice/non-lattice analysis requires the development of more efficient algorithms for non-lattice detection and extraction, which is covered in this chapter as well. Chapter 5 highlights the power and utility of uncovering non-lattice structures for debugging ontologies. Chapter 6 describes methods that leverage the linguistic information in concept names (labels) for ontological analysis. Chapter 7 addresses visualization and performance evaluation issues. Finally, Chap. 8 recaps the main message of the book and provides some forward-looking perspectives on the field. The appendix at the end of the book provides a list of key ontological resources, as well as annotated non-lattice and lattice examples that were actually discovered using our methods, demonstrating how "bugs are fixed" by converting non-lattices to lattices (with minimal edit changes).

Audience. The book is intended for graduate students and researchers interested in biomedical ontologies and their applications. It is more of a research monograph than a textbook. It can be used in conjunction with other materials for a course on biomedical ontologies or on knowledge representation and engineering. It can also serve as a reference to point the reader to related scientific publications and literature cited therein for identifying potential research topics. All mathematical concepts and notations used in this book can be found in standard Discrete Mathematics textbooks.

Houston, USA   Guo-Qiang Zhang
September 2022   Rashmie Abeysinghe
                                                                                        Licong Cui

Acknowledgements

The work presented in this book would not have been possible without the support and input from many collaborators and domain experts. First and foremost, we would like to express thanks to Olivier Bodenreider for his introduction to the field of biomedical ontologies and for being an inspiring collaborator. We thank our current and former research group members, Shiqiang Tao, Yan Huang, Xiaojin Li, Wei-chun Chou, Wei Zhu, Lingyun Luo, Fengbo Zheng, Qi Sun, Guangming Xing, Mengmeng Sun, and Songmao Zhang, for their contribution to the reported work. We thank the domain experts who provided feedback and contributed to the evaluation of the reported methods: Olivier Bodenreider, Samden Lhatoo, Jeffrey Talbert, Hunter Moseley, Eugene Hinderer, Jim Zheng, Yuntao Yang, Mason Bartels, Elmer Bernstam, James Case, Jay Shi, Cliff Joslyn, and Jose Mejino. We appreciate the encouragement and feedback from colleagues including Susan Redline, Yehoshua Perl, James Geller, Chunhua Weng, Tao Cui, Rong Xu, Guoqian Jiang, Mark Musen, and James Cimino.

We are grateful to our prior and current home institutions for providing supportive and nurturing environments for the research program that enabled this work: Case Western Reserve University, the University of Kentucky, and the University of Texas Health Science Center at Houston.

We are pleased to acknowledge that the research work reported here has been funded in part or in whole through awards from the National Institutes of Health (NIH) and the National Science Foundation (NSF). These include R01NS126690, R01NS116287, and U01NS090408 from the National Institute of Neurological Disease and Stroke (NINDS); R01LM013335 from the National Library of Medicine (NLM); R21CA231904 from the National Cancer Institute (NCI); R21AG068994 from National Institute on Aging (NIA); and R24HL114473 from the National Heart, Lung, and Blood Institute (NHLBI). Awards from the NSF division of Information and Intelligent Systems (IIS) include NSF-IIS 1657306, NSF-IIS 1931134, NSF-IIS 1816805, and NSF-IIS 2047001, and NSF Office of Advanced Cyberinfrastructure (OAC) NSF-ACI 1626364. The content of this book is solely the responsibility of the authors and does not necessarily represent the official views of the NSF or NIH.

We appreciate the continued encouragement and support from Series editors Ying Ding and Paul Groth, and from Morgan & Claypool Publishers' team led by Michael Morgan for making this book possible.

September 2022   Guo-Qiang Zhang
                                                                                            Rashmie Abeysinghe
                                                                                                     Licong Cui

Contents

About the Authors

Guo-Qiang Zhang is the inaugural holder of Distinguished Chair in Digital Innovation and a Professor of Medicine, Biomedical Informatics, and Public Health at the University of Texas Health Science Center at Houston (UTHealth Houston). He serves as co-director for the Texas Institute for Restorative Neurotechnologies and UTHealth's vice president and chief data scientist. Before joining UTHealth, he served as the inaugural director of the Institute for Biomedical Informatics, chief of the Division of Biomedical Informatics, and associate director of the Center for Clinical and Translational Science at the University of Kentucky. He spent prior years as faculty at the Case School of Engineering and School of Medicine at Case Western Reserve University, where he created its Division of Biomedical Informatics in the School of Medicine.

GQ Zhang received his Ph.D. in Computer Science from Cambridge University. His research spans large-scale, multi-center data integration, biomedical ontology development and quality assurance, clinical and research informatics, and agile, interface-driven, access-control-grounded software development. During the last decade, he led a research group that has developed production strength, informatics tools for data capturing, data management, cohort discovery, and clinical decision support, resulting in over 200 scientific publications and multiple awards across the National Institutes of Health (NIH) and the National Science Foundation (NSF).

Rashmie Abeysinghe is an Assistant Professor (Research) in the Department of Neurology at The University of Texas Health Science Center at Houston. He received his B.S. degree in Computer Science from the University of Peradeniy, Sri Lanka (2014) and Ph.D. degree in Computer Science from the University of Kentucky, USA (2020). He completed a Summer Internship at the National Library of Medicine, NIH in 2019. In 2020, he joined the Department of Neurology, McGovern Medical School at the University of Texas Health Science Center at Houston as a Research Scientist. His research interests revolve around biomedical ontologies, particularly from a quality assurance perspective, information extraction, and deep learning. His paper won a Distinguished Paper Award at the 2021 AMIA Annual Symposium. His papers were also selected as finalists for both the 2018 and 2019 AMIA Annual Symposium Student Paper Competitions.

Licong Cui received her Ph.D. in Computer Science from Case Western Reserve University (2014). She is an associate professor in the School of Biomedical Informatics at the University of Texas Health Science Center at Houston. Before joining UTHealth, she was an assistant professor in the Department of Computer Science and a member of the Institute for Biomedical Informatics at the University of Kentucky. Her research interests include ontologies and terminologies, neuroinformatics, big data analytics, large-scale data integration and management, and information extraction and retrieval. She has been a Principal Investigator of a number of highly competitive research awards funded by the NIH and the NSF. She is a recipient of the prestigious NSF CAREER Award and AMIA New Investigator Award.

Introduction

1.1 Biomedical Ontologies

It has been estimated that every two days, the human race is now generating as much data as were generated from the dawn of humanity through the year 2003 [1]. As scientific discovery today is being enabled through computational- and data-intensive research that exploits the enormous amounts of available data; this exponential growth fueled the rapid development of data science as a distinct discipline. Big data and the resurgence of machine learning, particularly in its recent incarnation of deep learning, highlight the importance of the availability of data and assurance of data quality as integral parts of efforts in advancing the frontiers of science, engineering, and biomedicine.

Ontologies are special types of data. They serve as metadata that can be used for the definition, annotation (labeling), indexing, linkage (mapping), extraction, integration, retrieval, enrichment, harmonization, and interaction of data. Ontologies, as shared conceptualization of a domain represented in a formal language, represent not only the concepts used in scientific work, but just as importantly, the relationships between the concepts. In biomedicine, the Unified Medical Language System (UMLS), produced and distributed by US National Library of Medicine (NLM), is the largest integrated repository of biomedical controlled vocabularies to facilitate interoperability among disparate systems in biomedicine and health. The source vocabularies include SNOMED CT US Edition (SNOMEDCT_US), SNOMED CT Spanish Language Edition (SCTSPA), Gene Ontology (GO), Foundational Model of Anatomy (FMA), Human Phenotype Ontology (HPO), and NCI Thesaurus (NCIt) [2].

Knowledge in the UMLS is presented in three categories: Metathesaurus, Semantic Network, and SPECIALIST Lexicon and Lexical Tools. The UMLS Metathesaurus is organized by concept (or meaning). Term variants from source vocabularies are clustered together to form a concept, and each concept is assigned a unique concept identifier (CUI). The basic building blocks (or atoms) of the UMLS Metathesaurus are the concept names or strings

G.-Q. Zhang et al., *Formal Methods for the Analysis of Biomedical Ontologies*,
Synthesis Lectures on Data, Semantics, and Knowledge,
https://doi.org/10.1007/978-3-031-12131-9_1

from each source vocabulary. Every occurrence of a concept name in each source is assigned a unique atom identifier (AUI) [2]. For instance, the concept names *"Hypertension,"* *"High blood pressure,"* and *"Hypertensive disorder"* from SNOMEDCT_US have AUIs A2882711, A2876587, and A3501627, respectively. *"Hypertension"* and *"Vascular Hypertensive Disorder"* from NCIt has AUIs A7571194 and A7628940, respectively. Concept names from different sources that represent the same meaning are assigned a unique CUI: C0020538. Moreover, relationships between concept terms in source vocabularies are preserved in the UMLS as relationship attributes. To give a sense of the size of UMLS, its 2015AB release contained over 3.2 million concepts and 12.8 million unique concept names from more than 190 source vocabularies.

In addition to standard ontological systems supported by government agencies and health organizations, the BioPortal of the National Center for Biomedical Ontology is the largest repository of ontologies generated by the biomedical research community [3, 4]. It also provides resources for ontology mapping, annotation, editing, and visualization. The Bio-Portal contains 960 ontologies from a range of domains, capturing 13.5 million classes, 36 thousand properties, and 55.65 million mappings.

1.1.1 Roles of Biomedical Ontologies

Ontologies serve as the semantic scaffolding for us to fully capitalize on the transformative opportunities of the increasingly large amounts of digital data produced by the biomedical research enterprise. Biomedical ontologies provide the basis for scientific rigor during the process of data collection, annotation, management, analysis, and sharing (Fig. 1.1). They not only serve as a part of the metadata standards for describing data in the FAIR Data Principles (Findable, Accessible, Interoperable, Reusable) [5], but also play a vital role in downstream systems as a declarative knowledge source. For example, SNOMED CT facilitates the clear exchange of health information in Electronic Health Records (EHRs), leading to higher quality, consistency and safety in healthcare delivery.

One can think of raw data, data dictionaries, common data elements, controlled terminologies, and ontologies as a cascading chain of digital resources of progressively higher conceptual degrees along the data-information-knowledge-wisdom (DIKW) hierarchy (Fig. 1.2) [6]. The DIKW hierarchy (other than wisdom) can be considered as data; there is value added in the direction of FAIRness when we link consecutive data entities in this cascading chain through analytics, annotation, and mapping. This strategy is expected to offer opportunities for new interfaces (for human or for machine) for data interpretability and integrability, leading to enhanced rigor and reproducibility.

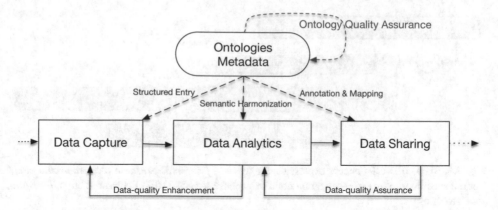

Fig. 1.1 Possible roles of ontologies in the data life cycle

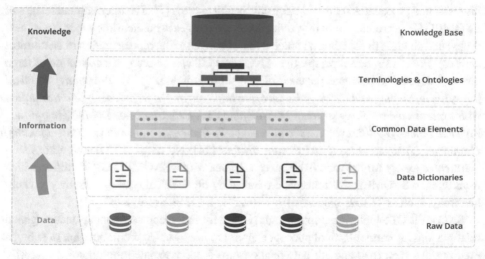

Fig. 1.2 Raw data, data dictionaries, common data elements, controlled terminologies, and ontologies along the DIKW hierarchy

1.1.2   SNOMED CT, Gene Ontology and NCI Thesaurus

The primary ontologies used in this book are SNOMED CT [7], GO [8] and NCIt [9]. Some chapters also use FMA [10].

SNOMED CT

Developed by the International Health Terminology Standard Development Organization (IHTSDO) and trading as SNOMED International [11], SNOMED CT is the world's largest clinical terminology [12]. It provides broad coverage of clinical medicine, including findings,

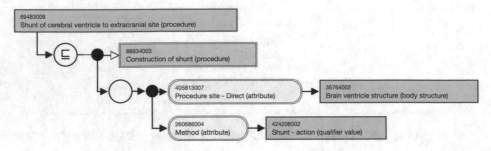

Fig. 1.3 SNOMED CT concept expression for *"Shunt of cerebral ventricle to extracranial site."* For the specific meaning of the diagram notations, please see SNOMED Browser at https://browser. ihtsdotools.org

diseases, and procedures for use in electronic health records [7]. The international release of SNOMED CT is produced monthly, reflecting both changes to medical knowledge (e.g., new drugs) and changes to the editorial process (e.g., changes to the representation of anatomical entities). From a structural perspective, SNOMED CT can be seen as a collection of large directed acyclic graphs, one for each of its "sub-hierarchies" [13]: *Procedure, Physical force, Event, Staging and scales, Substance, Environment or geographical location, Situation with explicit context, Body structure, Observable entity, Pharmaceutical/biologic product, Physical object, Qualifier value, Special concept, Specimen, Social context, Clinical finding, Organism, Linkage concept, and Record artifact* [14]. No concept is shared across sub-hierarchies except for the root. Each concept comes with a SNOMED CT identifier, which is an integer. SNOMED CT concepts are linked by hierarchical relations within each sub-hierarchy, such as *"Tissue specimen from heart" is-a "Tissue specimen"* [14].

SNOMED CT adopted description logic (DL) to formally represent concept meanings and relationships. A normal form of concept expression is a structured combination of subtype relationships (i.e., *is-a*) and attribute relationships (e.g., associated morphology, causative agent, finding site, part of) [15]. For example, the definition of *"Shunt of cerebral ventricle to extracranial site"* is shown in Fig. 1.3 using such a normal form [16].

Gene Ontology

The GO is a codified knowledge source for the unification of biology, widely adopted for codifying, managing, and sharing biological knowledge. GO provides a controlled vocabulary of terms for describing gene and gene product characteristics and related annotation data from GO Consortium members [8]. GO consists of a collection of three ontologies to describe attributes of gene products in three non-overlapping domains of molecular biology: *Cellular Component*, the parts of a cell or its extracellular environment; *Molecular Function*, the elemental activities of a gene product at the molecular level, such as binding or catalysis; and *Biological Process*, operations or sets of molecular events with a defined beginning and end, pertinent to the functioning of integrated living units (cells, tissues, organs, and organisms) [17]. Within each ontology, terms have free text definitions and unique identifiers. GO terms can be related to each other by relationships such as *is-a* and *part-of*, forming a directed acyclic graph. The GO vocabulary is designed to be species-agnostic, and is intended to capture multiple organisms [18].

NCI Thesaurus

The NCIt is a biomedical terminology for cancer research, covering vocabulary for clinical care, translational and basic research, and public information and administrative activities. It was first published in 2000 with the intention to facilitate data sharing and interoperability by different NCI centers and laboratories [19]. Concepts in NCIt are hierarchically organized in 19 domains, including *Abnormal Cell; Anatomic Structure, System, or Substance; Biological Process; Disease, Disorder or Finding; Drug, Food, Chemical or Biomedical Material; Gene, Gene Product, Molecular Abnormality*; and *Organism* [20]. The 22.04 d version of NCIt contains over 170,000 concepts. The NCIt was built using Ontylog, a description logic explicitly for building large complex terminologies. It is published in several formats including Ontylog XML, Web Ontology Language (OWL), and flat files [9]. The NCIt also has defined and inferred versions. The defined version contains the assertions about each concept by the terminology editors. The inferred version includes additional statements and classifications inferred by DL classifiers.

1.2   Structure and Definition

The principal components of an ontology are concepts and relations [21]. A "concept" represents a set of entities within a domain. For example, *"Protein"* is a concept within the domain of molecular biology referring to the set of all proteins. Relations describe the logical linkage between concepts or a concept's properties. In contrast to the mathematical notion of a set, defined by their extension (i.e. the entities that are part of the set), concepts in ontologies are defined "intensionally" by specifying their properties, features and relations that all the entities belonging to a concept must have (i.e., a logical definition).

A basic type of relation between concepts is the subclass (or *is-a*, or hierarchical) relationship. Using this subclass relationship, concepts in an ontology are typically organized into a hierarchy with more generic concepts modeled as parents of more specific concepts [22]. The subclass relationship serves to fixate the semantics of a concept precisely.

One can think of an ontology as a directed (multi-) graph or, sometimes more appropriately, a partially ordered set. Nodes in the graph correspond to concepts (or classes), and edges between nodes represent relations. Relations can be of different types, such as subclass (*is-a*), *part-of*, and *has-findingsite*. The *is-a* relation is considered the ontological backbone due to its fundamental role in classifying entities into subclasses. Intuitively, an ontology can be visualized or pictured as a "tree," with more general concepts appearing near the root, and more specialized concepts near the leaves for the subclass hierarchy. When rendering the *is-a* relations as a graph, the Hasse diagram convention [23] orients more general concepts above (or higher than) more specific concepts according to the notion of partially ordered set.

Indeed, the tree property, defined in the sense of mono-inheritance, or each node other than the root node has a unique parent, is sometimes adopted as a property of design (deliberately enforced), such as in the case of ICDs (9th or 10th edition) and MeSH. In general, however, multiple inheritance where a concept (node) many have multiple parents, is more natural and commonly seen in ontologies.

As can be seen from the rest of the book, ontological hierarchies determined by the *is-a* relation can exhibit more complex structural configurations such that they do not conform to tree or even lattice property, as often implicitly expected. To explain these points and fix notation for the rest of the book, recall that a partially ordered set (poset) is a set L with a reflexive, transitive relation $\leq \subseteq L \times L$. If $(L, \leq)$ is a poset, then its dual is the poset $(L, \geq)$ with the relation reversed. We denote posets by their carrier set as long as the partial order is clear from the context. An element u is called an *upper bound* of a subset $X \subseteq L$, if for each $x \in X$ we have $x \leq u$. For convenience, we write $\mathsf{ub}(X)$ for the set of upper bounds of X. An element m is called a *minimal upper bound* of a subset $X \subseteq L$, if m is an upper bound of X, and for any $n \leq m$ such that $x \leq n$ for each $x \in X$, we have $m = n$. We write $\mathsf{mub}(X)$ for the set of minimal upper bounds of X. When $\mathsf{mub}(X)$ is a singleton, the unique minimal upper bound is called the least upper bound, or join, of X. Dually, an element $l \in L$ is called a *lower bound* of a subset $X \subseteq L$, if for each $x \in X$ we have $x \geq l$. For convenience, we write $\mathsf{lb}(X)$ for the set of lower bounds of X. An element m is called a *maximal lower bound* (or meet) of a subset $X \subseteq L$, if m is a lower bound of X, and for any $n \geq m$ such that $x \geq n$ for each $x \in X$, we have $m = n$. We write $\mathsf{mlb}(X)$ for the set of maximal lower bounds of X. When $\mathsf{mlb}(X)$ is a singleton, the unique maximal lower bound is called the greatest lower bound, or meet, of X.

To illustrate these notions, we show some brief examples illustrated by Fig. 1.4. In Fig. 1.4, element 7 is an upper bound of $\{4, 5\}$. So is 8. Therefore, $\mathsf{ub}\{4, 5\} = \{7, 8\}$. Since 7 is the smallest element in $\mathsf{ub}\{4, 5\}$, it is a minimal upper bound. In fact, $\mathsf{mub}\{4, 5\} = \{7\}$, and so 7 is the join, or the least upper bound of the set $\{4, 5\}$. On the other hand, for the set $\{1, 2\}$, we have $\mathsf{mub}\{1, 2\} = \{6, 7\}$, i.e., the set $\{1, 2\}$ has two distinct minimal upper bounds (shaded light pink). The pair 1, 2 is called a *non-lattice* pair. Dually, the set $\{5, 6\}$ has a unique maximal lower bound, or meet, which is 2. On the other hand, the set $\{6, 7\}$ has two maximal lower bound, and we have $\mathsf{mlb}(\{6, 7\}) = \{1, 2\}$. Therefore, the pair 6, 7 does not have a meet.

A poset L is a *lattice* if every two elements of L have a join and a meet. These meets and joins of binary sets will be written in infix notation: $\bigvee\{x, y\} = x \vee y$ and $\bigwedge\{x, y\} = x \wedge y$. A poset L is a *complete lattice* if every subset $S \subseteq L$ has a least upper bound $\bigvee S$ (join) and a greatest lower bound (meet) $\bigwedge S$.

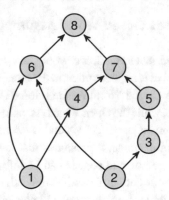

Fig. 1.4 A simple poset used to illustrate the order-theoretic notions, where $x \to y$ means $x \le y$

In connection with ontology, one can think of concepts as elements of a poset, and the ordering relation as the *is-a* subclass relation. In fact, the poset shown in Fig. 1.4 is exactly an ontological fragment from SNOMED CT, as illustrated in Fig. 1.5 (on the right). If x, y are concepts, we write $x \le y$ to mean x *is-a* y, or y subsumes x. In lattice-theoretic notation, the join $x \vee y$ of two concepts x, y is the lowest common ancestor of x and y, and the meet $x \wedge y$ is their greatest common descendant. For example, with respect to the poset in Fig. 1.4, we have $4 \vee 5 = 7$ and $5 \wedge 6 = 2$, although neither $1 \vee 2$ nor $6 \wedge 7$ exists.

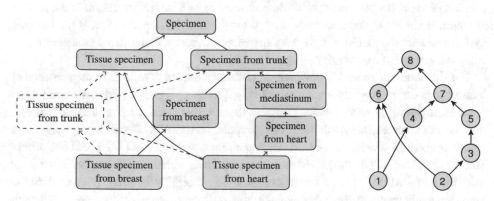

Fig. 1.5 Left: A non-lattice fragment in SNOMED CT (solid lines). Adding the dashed node and substituting the dashed edges for the solid edges to "*Tissue specimen*" would result in a lattice fragment. Right: abstracted version of the fragment on the left with node 1 for "*Tissue specimen from breast;*" 2 for "*Tissue specimen from heart;*" 3 for "*Specimen from heart;*" 4 for "*Specimen from breast;*" 5 for "*Specimen from mediastinum;*" 6 for "*Tissue specimen;*" 7 for "*Specimen from trunk;*" and 8 for "*Specimen.*"

1.2.1   Open-World Versus Closed-World Assumption

Though not often emphasized or clarified, we would like to make some of the working assumptions about biomedical ontologies explicit in the context of Open-World and Closed-World assumptions [24]. The Closed World Assumption (CWA) assumes that what is not known to be true must be false, while the Open World Assumption (OWA) assumes that what is not known to be true is simply unknown. CWA and OWA have important implications for knowledge representation. For example, it presumes that in a knowledgebase represented as logical statements, anything known to be true can be inferred from the knowledgebase. Therefore, anything that cannot be derived from the knowledgebase must be false. The OWA, on the other hand, presumes an incomplete, "open" knowledgebase, and does not make a commitment to the truth status of a statement when its truth cannot be determined based on inferences using existing facts in the knowledgebase.

When it comes to biomedical ontologies, which assumption, if any, is assumed? The answer is that mixed assumptions are used.

For the edge-relation, *is-a*, for example, CWA is implicitly assumed. For two concepts x and y in an ontology, if there is no *is-a* relation between the two (after inference using transitive closure), then we can safely assume that it is false to state that either x *is-a* y, or y *is-a* x, because otherwise the ontology would have modeled these as such, respectively. Continuing on the example earlier, the lack of an *is-a* edge between 1 and 2, "*Tissue specimen from breast*" and "*Tissue specimen from heart*," entails that a statement asserting an *is-a* relation between the two concepts would be known to be false (rather than unknown). This situation is similar to the commonly used airline booking system analogy: if the booking system does not show a direct flight from airport x to airport y, then there is indeed no direct flight connecting the two airports.

For the concepts, or nodes, however, an OWA is assumed. The lack of the presence of a concept in an ontology does not mean that such a concept does not exist, nor does it say anything about any possible relations between the concepts in the ontology and the concepts that are not captured in the ontology. For example, "*SARS-CoV-2*" was incorporated as a newer concept in several biomedical ontologies such as SNOMED CT (UMLS Concept Unique Identifier—CUI C5203676) more recently. Even with this addition, we still cannot infer from SNOMED CT that all descendants of the concept "*RNA virus*" (CUI C0035691) are completely captured. For concepts, the lack of their appearance does not entail their non-existence.

The real-world situation can sometimes be more nuanced. For example, for SNOMED CT, there is a distinction between "primitive concepts" and "fully-specified concepts." Intuitively, concepts labeled as primitive are intended to invoke an OWA with respect to relations involving them, while those labeled fully-specified invoke a CWA with respect to relations involving them. The gaps or editorial judgement inconsistencies between such intended designation (labeling) and the true status of affairs are often revealed by effective ontological analysis methods.

1.2.2   Properties of is-a and Other Ontological Principles

Cimino's famous "Desiderata" for controlled medical vocabularies put forth a list of ontology design guidelines required to serve their intended uses [25]. Among this list, *concept orientation, concept permanence, poly-hierarchy, and formal definitions* are prerequisites particularly relevant to the themes of this book. Concept orientation means that each concept has a single intended meaning, which needs to be taken for granted in order to subject them for analysis using formal methods. That this meaning, or semantics, is persistent and not drifted over time, is a requirement called concept permanence. Persistent, unambiguous semantics for concepts is achieved by placing them in rich enough context (or concept neighborhood), specified in their relationship to other concepts and even mappings to equivalent concepts in external ontologies. This highlights the need for us to consider relations (hierarchical *is-a* or otherwise) as first-class citizens in ontological modeling. Persistent, unambiguous semantics for concepts also requires the embracement of poly-hierarchy, or multiple-inheritance, and not to artificially enforce a tree structure just for the convenience of being able to perform "tree walking."

However, ontological structures should not be allowed to exhibit arbitrary complex structural properties (in the mathematical sense) either, and this book considers one additional item in the list of desiderata: that ontological hierarchies determined by the *is-a* relation should obey the lattice property. As can be seen in what follows, we may not want the "poly-hierarchy" to get too wild, beyond being lattices (see example earlier). Most of the subsequence development of our formal methods revolve around the topic of lattices vs non-lattices. Even though non-lattices—structures beyond or not conforming to lattices—are sometimes unavoidable in practice, they do represent more fruitful targets for "debugging." Therefore, the net effect of ontological quality enhancement may be measured by the reduction of non-lattice substructures.

Highly relevant to the formal methods theme of the book are a set of principles proposed by Bodenreider and Zhang [26], that is expected or should be enforced for well-formed ontologies. Many of the principles are examined in this book through explicit algorithms: they include the requirement that no hierarchical cycles are allowed and incompatible relationships (e.g., two concepts cannot be in relationship with two distinct relation-types).

1.2.3   Formal Concept Analysis, Lattices, and Non-lattices

Formal Concept Analysis (FCA) is a mathematical theory concerned with the formalization of concepts and conceptual thinking [27]. With FCA, we can generate a concept hierarchy from a collection of objects and attributes. The input of FCA is *formal context* $K = (O, A, R)$, where O is a set of objects, A is a set of attributes, and R is a binary relation between O and A. The notation $(o, a) \in R$ means that object o has attribute a.

Each formal context K induces two operators: derivation operators $\uparrow: 2^O \to 2^A$ and concept-forming operators $\downarrow: 2^A \to 2^O$. The operators are defined, for each $X \subseteq O$ and $Y \subseteq A$, as follows:

$$X^\uparrow = \{a \in A | \forall o \in X: (o, a) \in R\},$$

$$Y^\downarrow = \{o \in O | \forall a \in Y: (o, a) \in R\},$$

where $X^\uparrow$ is the set of all attributes shared by all objects in X, and $Y^\downarrow$ is the set of all objects sharing all attributes in Y.

A formal concept of K is a pair (X, Y) with $X \subseteq O$ and $Y \subseteq A$ such that $X^\uparrow = Y$ and $Y^\downarrow = X$. The subconcept-superconcept relation between formal concepts is given by $(X_1, Y_1) \le (X_2, Y_2)$ if and only if $X_1 \subseteq X_2 (Y_2 \subseteq Y_1)$. The fundamental theorem of FCA states that the collection of all formal concepts derived from a formal context K, under the subconcept-superconcept relation, always forms a complete lattice.

Lattices arise naturally from many disciplines. We speak of lattices because of their familiarity and their elegant structural properties. FCA offers mathematics support for lattice to be a desirable structural property for the taxonomy relation (*is-a*) in ontologies. Given the philosophical assumption that intension and extension are fundamental adjoining facets of the notion of *concept*, one can arrive at the mathematical structure of *(complete) lattices* automatically using FCA. Thus conformation to the lattice property is a powerful, universal ontological principle.

1.3   Ontological Analysis: Approaches

Given its size and complexity, it is unavoidable that errors and imperfections may exist in ontologies as a part of its development, update, and maintenance lifecycle. It is impractical for domain experts to uncover potential errors and inconsistencies based on exhaustive manual review. Automatic and effective approaches to quality assurance are highly desirable, moving domain experts' role towards review and confirmation of automatically discovered error candidates. Ideally, each error discovered comes with an automatically generated change suggestion, so that correction of these errors are greatly facilitated and incorporated in subsequent versions.

Researchers have proposed lexical, structural, and semantic methods for auditing and quality improvement of biomedical terminologies and ontologies. Several survey papers provide a valuable overview of the state of the art of methods for ontological analysis. Themes of the surveys include auditing methods applied to the content of controlled biomedical terminologies [28], auditing techniques specifically applied for the Unified Medical Language System [29], and ontology evaluation practice in the biomedicine domain [30].

The general pipeline of ontological analysis (including auditing, quality assurance, and evaluation) involves fives steps, as shown in Fig. 1.6.

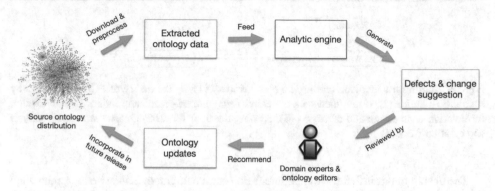

Fig. 1.6 The general pipeline of ontological analysis: Step 1-Download and preprocess an ontology to obtain data in an analyzable format; Step 2-Feed the preprocessed data into an analytic engine (e.g., auditing algorithm, quality assurance, and evaluation tools); Step 3-Produce output capturing the results of the analysis in a format that domain experts and ontological engineers can make sense of (e.g., suitable graphical rendering); Step 4-Evaluate the results and translate the findings into specific actionable suggestions; Step 5-Make change recommendations to the ontology owner for possible adoption into future releases

Many existing methods lack attention for steps 3, 4, and 5, particularly in their ability to pinpoint possible errors and suggest remedies, rather than merely identifying "potential problem areas" or "likely issues." This is also why evaluation alone, using some predefined metric, statistics or scoring system, does not automatically lead to quality enhancement outcomes.

We argue that to qualify as "formal methods," a method must be able, at least in principle, to address all these five steps in Fig. 1.6. As can be seen from the rest of the book, methods described here are illustrated for their abilities to pinpoint potential errors and suggest change remedies. In particular, we leverage the lattice property as a guiding principle in locating specific inconsistencies and errors. The deeper philosophical and mathematical reason for lattice to be a desirable structural property for the *is-a* relation in ontologies can be elucidated with FCA. Starting from two very basic sets—objects and attributes—one always obtains a (complete) lattice automatically (Fig. 1.7) using FCA.

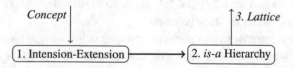

Fig. 1.7 With the assumption that intension and extension are fundamental adjoining facets of the notion of concept (1), one can derive a concept hierarchy (2) which is guaranteed by the mathematical theory of FCA to be a lattice (3)

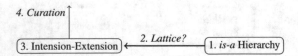

Fig. 1.8 Starting from a given ontological *is-a* hierarchy (1), by the theory of FCA, this hierarchy should be a lattice (2). If not, then such a hierarchy may not be completely induced by an explicit formulation of intension and extension (3), opening the door for error-agnostic structural analysis and curation work (4)

The upshot of this is that if we encounter a non-lattice fragment in the *is-a* hierarchy, then there could be one or multiple sources of error that contributing to it. For example, redundant concepts can manifest themselves as multiple minimal upper bounds. If *is-a* relationship is used too liberally where in fact *part-of* relationship should be used, this can also easily introduce non-lattice fragments. If the notion of intension and extension associated with the concepts changes from an area in the ontology to another, then the resulting concept hierarchy may violate the lattice property as well. The most common reason for non-lattice fragments to arise is due to "semantic incompleteness" or "inconsistency in pre-coordination." All of these anomalies can be difficult to detect otherwise (Fig. 1.8).

1.3.1 Evaluation on Performance of Analytical Methods

Debugging for software defects is like finding needles in a haystack. Finding ontological errors (anomalies, inconsistencies, or incompleteness) is similar in spirit.

In this context, it is unreasonable to expect 100% precision or 100% recall in finding all ontological defects. In fact, the nature of the task should be more appropriately compared to finding gold mine or oil fields. It is logically impossible to assess recall in the absolute sense, because "ground truth" simply does not exist: an exhaustive list of all the true errors is unattainable due to the fundamental nature of the topic of study. Lower precision should also be acceptable, because validated errors can cumulate and result in enhanced future releases of ontologies.

In reality, evaluation of methods for ontology analysis, if they are incorporated in a study, inevitably involve manual work by domain experts. To be feasible, evaluations are performed on only a sample of randomly selected results.

This is in sharp contrast to the performance evaluation on machine learning or deep learning models, where precision and recall lower than 80% are simply not viewed as competitive.

1.3.2   Interactability with Ontologies: Search and Visualization

Ontology query and visualization is essential to facilitate sophisticated quality assurance work in ontological evolution. Visualization tools for ontologies have been developed for viewing terminology content or hierarchy structure. The official *SNOMED Browser* is a web-based, multilingual, multi-edition ontology browsing application [16]. It enables browsing of International Edition of SNOMED CT, as well as various National Editions. Users can enter terms or navigate in the taxonomy hierarchies to find the target concept, with filters. The application provides the details of concepts, including descriptions, parents and children, attributes and structural diagrams.

Protégé is one of the most widely used ontology development tools [31]. Its framework allows interactive creation and visualization of classes in a hierarchical view. Particularly, *Protégé* is extendable via plug-ins, enabling developers to add additional functionality into the *Protégé* system. *Web-Protégé* is a web-based version of *Protégé* that focuses on collaborative ontology development. *OntoViz* is a *Protégé* plug-in to display an ontology as a 2D graph with the capability of showing the names, properties, inheritance, and relations [32]. *TGVizTab* visualizes *Protégé* ontologies in the spring layout where nodes repel one another, whereas the edges (links) attract them [33]. It allows users to navigate gradually making visible parts of the graph. Users may also perform expanding, retracting, hiding, and zooming operations to interact with the graph. *SHriMP* is a domain-independent visualization technique designed to enhance how people browse and explore complex information spaces [34]. *SHriMP* uses a nested graph view and supports concept navigation. One can expand the hierarchy graph by clicking the concept, which provides an intuitive visualization of its relationships. *Jambalaya* is a *Protégé* plug-in based on *SHriMP* with the enhancement of advanced keyword search, allowing users to search the whole ontology or limit the search scope by specifying the type of the searched item [35]. *OntoRama* is an ontology browser for RDF models based on a hyperbolic layout of nodes and arcs [36]. *OntoSphere* is a 3D tool that uses three different ontology views in order to provide an overview or detailed features, such as ancestors, children, and semantic relations [37]. *OAF* is a unified framework and software system for deriving, visualizing, and exploring partial-area taxonomy abstraction networks [38].

In general, sensemaking of ontological structures using proper visualization techniques is an important activity in ontological engineering. Graphical sensemaking of ontologies is the process of visualizing, exploring, and studying specific understandable substructures of a large ontological structure in order to reveal novel substructures of potential interest in a specific ontology. Making sense of ontological knowledge graphs can be a challenging but indispensable process of our intellectual enquiry, particularly for biomedical ontologies that are intended to capture the current state of knowledge in a domain. Even though global graph properties (e.g. distribution of the numbers of siblings of concepts, and concept density and balances) may not necessarily be directly relevant to sensemaking, they may play essential roles in the development of sensemaking systems with respect to optimized design of indices, graph query languages, and statistical summarization.

We consider the following as a basic set of requirements for graph visualization to be effective in supporting sensemaking of ontological structures:

1. The rendered ontological graph substructure must be of manageable size (at least four concepts should be included, however) in that concept nodes and edges are properly displayed and readable within the rendering window;
2. The substructure of potential interest can be effectively and dynamically allocated using search and information retrieval techniques;
3. The rendered substructure should be a faithful, complete representation of available information around the concepts and relations involved, i.e., it represents an embedded substructure and not merely an ontological subgraph. This allows the invocation of CWA for the rendered substructure by the user;
4. The rendering method should conform to the convention of Hasse Diagram, a standard rendering strategy for partially ordered sets displayed using the cover relation of the partially ordered set with an implied upward orientation.

As can be seen throughout the book, as well as in the appendix, we use graph rendering techniques for the visualization of lattice and non-lattice fragments in ontologies, conforming to the Hasse diagram convention, for ontology sensemaking and error discovery.

Simple Relational Patterns

This chapter describes methods to compare simple relational patterns during the evolution of an ontology (*is-a* reversal), detecting redundant hierarchical relations within the same ontology (existence of two distinct paths between a pair of concepts), mixed redundant patterns in the existence of two different types of relational paths between a pair of concepts, and comparing such simple patterns across ontologies. All of these "patterns" represent undesired artifact which should be examined closely or completely eliminated if possible.

2.1   Reversals

The focus of this section is on ontology evolution [39, 40], most specifically on hierarchical relation reversals in SNOMED CT. A simple example of such a reversal consists of two concepts: "*Joint structure of shoulder girdle*" and "*Joint structure of shoulder region.*" The 07/2013 version states that "*Joint structure of shoulder girdle*" *is-a* "*Joint structure of shoulder region,*" although the (more recent) 03/2014 version asserts the opposite (first two components in Fig. 2.1): "*Joint structure of shoulder region*" *is-a* "*Joint structure of shoulder girdle.*"

This is an example of a *direct (hierarchical relation) reversal*: "*A is-a B*" in one version has been changed to "*B is-a A*" in another version. An *indirect (hierarchical relation) reversal*, considered in this section, may involve *an arbitrary number of steps* in an entire path: $A \rightarrow^* B$ in one version is changed to $B \rightarrow^* A$ in another version, where $\rightarrow^*$ represents several *is-a* steps in the same direction. We call the concepts A and B involved in either a direct or an indirect relation reversal *a reversal pair*.

The purpose of this study is twofold: (1) Relation reversals represent an important and rather dramatic structural change, because all the parents and children of the reversed concepts are also affected. There may be good reasons for the occurrence of such reversals that could provide us insight for improving concept labels that better reflect the intended

G.-Q. Zhang et al., *Formal Methods for the Analysis of Biomedical Ontologies*,
Synthesis Lectures on Data, Semantics, and Knowledge,
https://doi.org/10.1007/978-3-031-12131-9_2

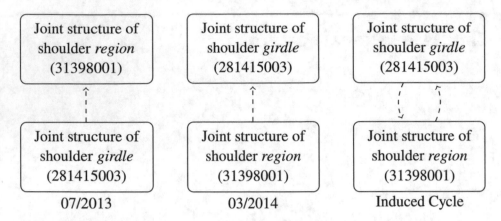

Fig. 2.1 First two arrows: reversal of *is-a* relation between two versions of SNOMED CT. Right most: a cycle induced by the reversal pair when it appears in a merged graph. The numbers below concept labels are the corresponding SNOMED CT identifiers

meaning. (2) Relation reversals are important for identifying and handling cycles for comparative visualization of ontological evolution. A common, perhaps most effective, tool for rendering directed acyclic graphs in general and hierarchical relations in ontological structures in particular, is topological sort (a.k.a. Coffman-Graham algorithm). Topological sort enables each concept assigned a unique *level*, followed by edge rendering. We are interested in visualizing ontological changes in such a way that two related fragments from different versions of the same ontology are *merged* into a single graph for visual inspection of the changes (Fig. 2.2). However, if a reversal pair is involved (Fig. 2.1, right most), it causes the merged graph cyclic, making topological sort not directly applicable. By identifying and handling reversals (the only source for introducing cycles) ahead of rendering, topological sort can still be utilized.

Mining all reversals (not just the direct ones) and between all SNOMED CT versions (not just the consecutive versions), is a computationally intensive task. We present a "Big Data" approach using MapReduce to systematically extract all such reversals among 8 SNOMED CT versions from 2009 to 2014.

2.1.1   MapReduce Approach for Reversal Detection

Our data source consists of 8 versions of SNOMED CT, dated 07/2009, 01/2010, 01/2011, 01/2012, 07/2012, 01/2013, 07/2013, and 03/2014. To detect direct and indirect hierarchical reversals among these versions of SNOMED CT, we first compute the transitive closure for each version based on the direct *is-a* relationship. Hierarchical relation reversals are then detected by set operations of the respective transitive closures using MapReduce. If all reversal pairs are direct reversals for these 8 versions, we would like to confirm so; but it

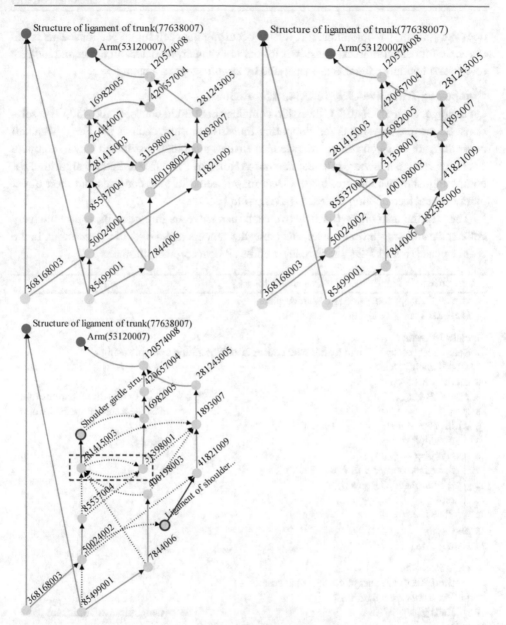

Fig. 2.2 Semi-automatically rendered graphs from two SNOMED CT versions. Top-left: a non-lattice fragment of 7/2013 version of SNOMED CT. Top-right: a non-lattice fragment of 03/2014 version of SNOMED CT. Bottom: merged graph showing the changes. The loop inside dotted red rectangle is caused by the reversal given in Fig. 2.1

does not rule out possible indirect reversals occurring between future versions. This is the rationale for using (indirect) transitive closure, to exhaustively detect all direct and indirect reversals, including pairs that are separated by several steps in a path.

Computing Transitive Closure Using MapReduce

On average, each SNOMED CT version contains about 300k concepts and 450k *is-a* relations. Sequential algorithms for computing transitive closure, such as the Floyd-Warshall algorithm, are time-consuming. MapReduce enables a parallel, distributed way to compute transitive closure in a more efficient manner. Algorithm 1 is our MapReduce algorithm for computing transitive closure. First, a hash map is setup to load concepts and their direct parents in each computing node using $DistributedCache$.

Then, in the map phase (lines 3–16), each mapper reads in a concept, and recursively collects its ancestors level by level, and emits the concept and the set of its ancestors. In the reduce phase (lines 17–21), each reducer emits all concept-ancestor pairs.

Algorithm 1: MapReduce for Transitive Closure

Input: Concept nodes and *is-a* relation pairs
Output: Transitive closure concept pairs

1 **class** MAPPER
2 Setup a HashMap CP and load it with concepts and their direct parents using $DistributedCache$.
3 **method** MAP(concept c)
4 $P = CP$.get(c)   ▷ Get direct parents of c
5 $A = \emptyset$ ▷ Initialize a set for ancestors of c
6 **while** $P \neq \emptyset$ **do**
7 $\quad$ A.add(P)
8 $\quad$ $temp = \emptyset$
9 $\quad$ **for** each concept p in P **do**
10 $\quad\quad$ $temp$.add(CP.get(p))
11 $\quad$ **end**
12 $\quad$ $P = temp$
13 **end**
14 EMIT(c, A)

15 **class** REDUCER
16 **method** REDUCE(concept c, concept ancestors A)
17 **for** each concept a in A **do**
18 $\quad$ EMIT(c, a)   ▷ Output transitive closure pairs
19 **end**

Algorithm 2: MapReduce Set Operations for Reversal

Input: Transitive closure concept pairs for two versions O and N
Output: Direct and indirect reversals between O and N

1 **class** MAPPER
2 **method** MAP(concept c_1, concept c_2)
3 **if** *the concept pair (c_1, c_2) is in O* **then**
4 | EMIT((c_1, c_2), O)
5 **else if** *the concept pair (c_1, c_2) is in N* **then**
6 | EMIT((c_2, c_1), N)   ▷ Reverse the concept pair in N

7 **class** REDUCER
8 **method** REDUCE((c_1, c_2), versions V)
9 **if** $|V| = 2$ **then**   ▷ The concept pair is in both O and reversed N
10 | EMIT(c_1, c_2)
11 **end**

Performing Big-Set-Operations Using MapReduce

Using the computed transitive closures for each SNOMED CT version, reaching over 5 million edges each, we detect reversals between any two versions by intersecting concept pairs in one version and reversed concept pairs in the other version.

Formally, given O and N, transitive closures for two SNOMED CT versions, the set of reversals between them is $\{(c_1, c_2) \mid (c_1, c_2) \in O\} \cap \{(c_2, c_1) \mid (c_1, c_2) \in N\}$.

This involves big-set-intersection, since transitive closure for each version contains a large number of concept pairs and traditional way of performing set operations does not always fit into memory. Therefore, we perform big-set-intersections in a more feasible and efficient way using MapReduce. Algorithm 2 shows the MapReduce algorithm to perform big-set-intersections and detect reversals between any two SNOMED CT versions. In the map stage (lines 3–9), each mapper reads in a set of concept pairs, and emits key-value pairs $((c_1, c_2), O)$ if the concept pair (c_1, c_2) is in O, and $((c_2, c_1), N)$ if the concept pair (c_1, c_2) is in N. In the reduce stage (lines 10–14), each reducer aggregates versions involved for a concept pair, and emits the concept pair if it belongs to both versions.

2.1.2   Reversals Identified in SNOMED CT and Utilization of the Method in Ontology Fragment Visualization

This section summarizes the results obtained with this approach. For detailed explanation about the method and the discussion about the results, please see [41].

Relation Reversals

We performed 28 pairwise comparisons among the 8 SNOMED CT versions and found 48 reversals (Table 2.1). Among the 48 reversals, 33 were from the sub-hierarchy Clinical Finding, 8 from Body Structure, 6 from Procedure, and 1 from Event. Two of the reversals (rows 07/2009 → 03/2014 and 01/2010 → 07/2013 in Table 2.1) had intermediate stages in

Table 2.1 Distribution of relation reversals in SNOMED CT sub-hierarchies and the versions in which they occurred. C: Clinical Finding. B: Body Structure. P: Procedure. E: Event

Version pair	C	B	P	E
07/2009 → 01/2010	7	0	2	0
01/2010 → 01/2011	7	0	3	0
01/2011 → 01/2012	7	0	0	0
01/2012 → 07/2012	0	0	0	0
07/2012 → 01/2013	1	0	0	0
01/2013 → 07/2013	1	0	0	0
07/2013 → 03/2014	9	7	1	1
07/2009 → 03/2014	0	1	0	0
01/2010 → 07/2013	1	0	0	0
Total (**48**)	33	8	6	1

which the pair is not coupled by an *is-a* relation, confirming our strategy to perform all 28 pairwise comparisons rather than performing comparison only for 7 consecutive versions.

Ten sample reversal pairs are displayed in Fig. 2.3. On average, computing the transitive closure of an entire SNOMED CT version and computing big-set-intersection between transitive closures each took less than 40 s, amounting to a total computing time of 18 min.

1. Premature or threatened labor (287979001), Premature labor (6383007);
2. Anesthesia for procedure on head and neck (82973008), Anesthesia for procedure on head (120212000);
3. Primary dilated cardiomyopathy (195021004), Primary idiopathic dilated cardiomyopathy (53043001);
4. Computed tomography of shoulder (241564007), Computed tomography arthrogram of shoulder (241583000);
5. Musculoskeletal structure of sacral spine (297169002), Sacral spine (303950008);
6. Rupture of tendon of biceps, long head (86128003), Rupture of tendon of biceps (428883008);
7. Joint structure of shoulder girdle (281415003), Joint structure of shoulder region (31398001);
8. Calcium deposits in tendon (404224009), Osteodesmosis (404225005);
9. Sciatic neuropathy (52585001), Sciatic nerve lesion (367137004);
10. Fly bite (283345006), Mosquito bite (283344005).

Fig. 2.3 10 sample reversal pairs among the result of 48

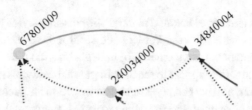

Fig. 2.4 Two pairs of indirect reversals. One pair consists of "*Tendinitis AND/OR tenosynovitis*" (240034000) and "*Inflammatory disorder of tendon*" (34840004); the other pair consists of "*Tendinitis AND/OR tenosynovitis*" (240034000) and "*Tenosynovitis*" (67801009)

Indirect Reversals

We found 12 indirect reversals. All such pairs involved one direct *is-a* relation in one version and a length-two path in the other version. Figure 2.4 shows 2 such indirect reversals. This confirms the validity of our strategy to compute transitive closures of SNOMED CT versions, because using the direct relations alone would have missed such reversals.

Our exhaustive analysis using transitive closure also assured that no reversals involving a path-length of more than 2 existed for the versions we analyzed. However, this does not rule out the existence of indirect reversals involving longer paths between future versions.

Enabling Visualization of Merged Fragments from Distinct SNOMED CT Versions

Our work on detecting direct and indirect reversals is also motivated by removing a technical barrier in visualizing merged ontological fragments from distinct versions of SNOMED CT. Ontological fragments in SNOMED CT can be visualized using SVG (scalable vector graphics - see Fig. 2.2), supported by common web browsers using the D3 drawing library (http://www.d3js.org). By convention, nodes represent concepts and edges represent *is-a* relation between concepts, with edge direction going from child (lower) to parent (higher). A well-known rendering algorithm for directed acyclic graphs is based on topological sort. We use this algorithm to render merged non-lattice fragments from different versions of SNOMED CT. However, relation reversals introduce cycles, making topological sort non-terminating. Thus detecting reversals before applying topological sort is required.

Figure 2.2 illustrates an example of a semi-automatically generated merged graph of two non-lattice fragments from Sect. 4.2 in distinct SNOMED CT versions. The fragments are generated from Body Structure concepts "*Arm*" (53120007) and "*Structure of ligament of trunk*" (77638007) in 01/2013 and 03/2014 versions of SNOMED CT. The loop (inside the red dotted rectangle) in the graph involves the reversal pair (item 7 in Fig. 2.3) of "*Joint structure of shoulder girdle*" (281415003) and "*Joint structure of shoulder region*" (31398001).

For Fig. 2.2, the source concept pair is colored in green. Nodes representing the greatest common descendants of the source pair are painted in yellow. All nodes lying in-between a green node and a yellow node appear in light gray. Additional graphical elements are used for visualizing graph changes (for both Figs. 2.2 and 2.4): red represents deletion and blue insertion. Nodes and edges are also marked with distinct styles to represent additional information: (a) nodes with solid red borders and solid red edges represent deletion: they appear in the old fragment but not the new; (b) nodes with solid blue borders and solid blue edges represent addition: they appear in the new fragment but not old; (c) nodes with dashed borders, and edges drawn in dashed style represent insertion and deletion in the SNOMED CT versions (such changes must appear in the respective fragments).

For further details and discussions about the technicalities of the non-lattice visualization system, please see Sect. 7.1.

2.1.3 Further Findings of the Method

Clinically, hierarchical relation reversals may involve concepts whose positions in the hierarchical structure are not immediately obvious. Concepts that are the object of relation reversals during ontological evolution may be worth further analysis (such as items 7 to 10 in Table 2.3). A majority of the reversals are consistent with two prior studies on the use of "and" and "or" [42] as well as "lexically assign, logically refine" [43].

And/Or
We found 18 reversal pairs involved the connectives "and" and "or" (or implicit logical conjunction, e.g., anorectal). For example (see items 1 and 2 in Table 2.3), "Premature or threatened labor, Premature labor" and "Anesthesia for procedure on head and neck, Anesthesia for procedure on head" are reversal pairs that represent a common possible misinterpretation of "and," which uses intersection in form to represent union in meaning. To make the intended meaning clearer, it is perhaps helpful to normalize the connective to "AND/OR" when the intended meaning is union, especially with respect to Body Structure and Procedure. With this convention, a concept in the form of A should always be a subclass of a concept of the form A AND/OR B. Further, all concepts "A and B" should be normalized to "A AND/OR B," so "Anesthesia for procedure on head and neck" should be normalized to "Anesthesia for procedure on head AND/OR neck" to avoid potential confusion. This is consistent with the analysis given in [42].

Lexically Assign, Logically Refine
Examples due to this type of phenomenon include the pairs in items 3, 4, 5, and 6 in Table 2.3. The lexicographical difference between the pairs involves the insertion of words, such as "idiopathic" in item 3, "arthrogram" in item 4, "Musculoskeletal structure of" in item 5, and "long head" in item 6. It is arguable that any such insertion of words results in a more specialized concept, and hence should be a subclass of the parent concept. However, in the latest version we analyzed (3/2014), the opposite seems to be the case sometimes. Further consideration is needed to come up with a guiding principle (rule) that can be systematically applied.

Big Data Approach for Ontology Quality Assurance Work

We consider *"Big Data" as a frame of mind, or a "bigger vision,"* in perceiving the scientific landscape from a grander data scale, emboldened by the scalability of cloud computing, such as MapReduce for massive parallel processing. Such an approach can dramatically accelerate the speed of analysis in cases of complex tasks that are less computationally feasible. We believe that such a scalable approach is beneficial for ontology quality assurance work in general, even for computationally feasible problems (such as the work presented here), because it allows us to ask bigger questions and to answer them faster, putting computational barrier on the back of our minds so we can focus more on the scientific content.

Conclusion: We presented a scalable and generalizable method using MapReduce to mine reversals during ontological evolution. 48 hierarchical reversals have been found in 8 SNOMED CT versions from 2009. Identification of such reversals allowed avoidance of cycles in applying topological sort for rendering merged ontological graphs for visual comparison and change illustration. The reversals confirmed prior findings in the literature about concept labeling convention recommendations, but also revealed new cases for further consideration. In general, our closure-based technique has shown to be powerful and efficient for analyzing large ontological structures as well as their evolution. Although this investigation focused on hierarchical reversals, our approach suggests the exploration of reversals of other kinds of relations, which we plan to address in future work.

2.2   Redundancy Detection

This section focuses on a particular type of ontological structural defect: redundant relations. Redundant hierarchical relations refer to such patterns as two paths from concept X to concept Y, one with length one (direct) and the other with length greater than one (indirect). For hierarchical relations such as subsumption (*is-a*), relations implied by transitivity should not be explicitly stated. For example, in Gene Ontology (GO 2015-05-01 version) we have (see Table 2.2):

Table 2.2 A = *"hormone secretion;"* B = *"hormone transport;"* C = *"regulation of hormone levels;"* D = *"regulation of biological quality;"* E = *"biological regulation;"* F = *"biological process"*

	GO Id	Relation		GO Id
A	GO:0046879	is-a	B	GO:0009914
B	GO:0009914	is-a	C	GO:0010817
C	GO:0010817	is-a	D	GO:0065008
D	GO:0065008	is-a	E	GO:0065007
E	GO:0065007	is-a	F	GO:0008150

Fig. 2.5 Graphical rendering
of Table 2.2 and a direct edge
between A and F. Directed
edges represent *is-a* relation

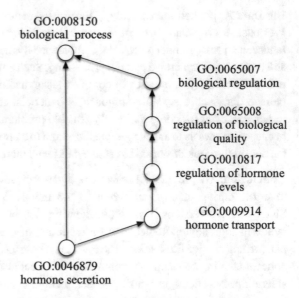

GO:0008150
biological_process

GO:0065007
biological regulation

GO:0065008
regulation of biological
quality

GO:0010817
regulation of hormone
levels

GO:0009914
hormone transport

GO:0046879
hormone secretion

However, "A (GO:0046879) *is-a* F (GO:0008150)" is directly asserted as well (Fig. 2.5).
This represents redundant relations to be studied in this section: two paths exist between
A and F: one directly between A and F, and the other indirectly through B, C, D, and E as
intermediate concept nodes.

The principle of parsimony in ontological modeling refers to the omission of relations
implied by the transitive property of a relationship, such as *is-a* relations in GO. By violating this principle, redundant relations may increase maintenance burden for ontology
curators. It can also cause inaccurate methods and algorithms based on this general principle. For example, semantic distance between concepts is a widely used technique [44].
Ontological mapping and alignment methods rely on the ordered structure of the hierarchical
relation [45], with notions of neighborhood and proximity serving as their foundation. The
presence of redundant relations induces a short-circuit: two concepts with a larger semantic
distance may result in a smaller distance by mistake; and concepts not within a neighborhood
may be counted as such.

Using brute force, exhaustive detection of redundant relations can be computationally
expensive for large ontologies. For example, SNOMED CT (2015-03-01 version) contains
over 300,000 active concepts. A naive approach would be to find the longest paths between
the end nodes of each of the over 500,000 edges (relations). *Assuming each edge takes*
100 ms, processing a single version of SNOMED CT would take 14 h. Finding all paths
between all possible pairs among the 300k nodes would take over 10,000 days if each pair
takes 10 ms.

Table 2.3 Summary of the results for 5 versions of SNOMED CT. TC: number of transitive closure pairs, RR: number of redundant *is-a* relations, T (ms): time taken in milliseconds

Version	# Concepts	# *is-a* Relations	TC	RR	RR%	T (ms)
2013-09-01	300,485	447,442	5,226,630	240	0.00459	10,472
2014-03-01	300,409	446,603	5,188,221	277	0.00534	10,335
2014-09-01	302,902	449,564	5,222,506	305	0.00584	10,074
2015-03-01	315,904	467,799	5,408,010	235	0.00435	15,264
2015-09-01	320,911	476,226	5,511,334	372	0.00675	16,077

This section introduces a novel and scalable approach, called FEDRR – Fast, Exhaustive Detection of Redundant Relations – for quality assurance work during ontological evolution. In contrast to the 14h naive approach required for each SNOMED CT version, *FEDRR needed < 20 s* (see Table 2.3).

2.2.1 Scalable Redundancy Detection Algorithm

The general mathematical abstraction of an ontological structure is a graph-theoretic one: nodes correspond to concepts, and edges correspond to relations (between nodes). For hierarchical relations in ontological systems such as *is-a*, which obeys the *transitivity property* that

$$\text{if } A \text{ is-a } B \text{ and } B \text{ is-a } C, \text{ then } A \text{ is-a } C,$$

one can model the structure of an ontological system as a directed acyclic graph (DAG, as shown in part in Fig. 2.5).

Definition 2.1 Suppose $G = (V, E)$ is a directed acyclic graph with V a set of nodes, and E a set of edges between the nodes. A redundant relation in G is a pair of nodes (s, t) such that $(s, t) \in E$, and there is an indirect path (i.e., length more than 1) from s to t.

The closely related known algorithm for computing redundant relations in the literature is all-pair longest path [46]. Although fixed source longest path can be solved in time-complexity $O(|V| + |E|)$ in a DAG [46], all-pair longest path requires iteration over V, resulting in an $O(|V| \cdot |E| + |V|^2)$ time-complexity algorithm.

Fig. 2.6 Basic mechanism for updating the D-set and the I-set of a node

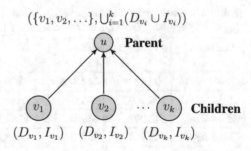

For large ontological systems such as SNOMED CT, such a running time amounts to an intractable amount of processing time (requiring 10,000 days if all-pair paths were to be computed).

FEDRR solves this problem in time-complexity $O(c \cdot |V| + |E|)$, where c is the average number of descendants of a node. For the latest version of SNOMED CT, we have $c = 17.12$ (see Time Complexity Analysis). For a single version of SNOMED CT, the actual processing time is less than $20\,s$.

There are two key algorithmic ideas behind FEDRR. One is avoidance of repeated computations by remembering the set of directly reachable nodes as well as the set of indirectly reachable nodes, for each node. The second is to completely skip node pairs that are not connected by a directed path. These ideas are reflected in FEDRR using a novel combination of dynamic programming with topological sort. The sparsity of most ontological structures, viewed as a DAG, is a particularly suitable property for the second idea to take advantage of.

For a node u in a DAG $G = (V, E)$, we introduce two sets, D_u and I_u, where

- $D_u = \{v \mid (v, u) \in E\}$, called the D-**set**, consists of the direct descendants (i.e., children) of u; and
- I_u, called the I-**set** of u, is the set of all indirect descendants of u.

The design of our algorithm is based on the following observation.

Lemma 2.2 *For each node $v \in D_u \cap I_u$, (v, u) is redundant.*

Algorithm 3: FEDRR: Dynamic programming using topological sort to compute the D-set and I-set of each node

---

1 **Input:** $G(V)$
2 $q := new\ Queue()$
3 **forall the** $v \in V$ **do**
4     $I[v] := \emptyset$
5     $D[v] := \emptyset$
6   **if** *no incoming edge for v* **then**
7         $q.enqueue(v)$
8   **end**
9 **end**
10 **while** *q not empty* **do**
11     $s := q.dequeue()$
12   **forall the** $t \in s.to$ **do**
13         $I[t] := I[t] \cup I[s] \cup D[s]$
14         $D[t] := D[t] \cup \{s\}$
15   mark edge (s, t)
16   **if** *no unmarked incoming edge for t* **then**
17             $q.enqueue(t)$
18   **end**
19   **end**
20 **end**

Our algorithm amounts to the computation of (D_u, I_u) for each node u. To utilize the idea of dynamic programming, we update (D_u, I_u) for each node u according to the order by topological sort. The basic update scheme is illustrated in the following diagram:

Suppose we have obtained (D_{v_i}, I_{v_i}) for each $i = 1, \ldots, k$, where $\{v_1, v_2, \ldots\} = \{v \mid (v, u) \in E\}$. Then we set $D_u = \{v_1, v_2, \ldots\}$ and $I_u = \bigcup_{i=1}^{k}(D_i \cup I_i)$. The pseudo-code of FEDRR appears in Algorithm 3.

FEDRR starts by initializing an empty queue to hold the nodes that will be sorted (line 2). Then nodes with no incoming edges are put to the queue, with the D-set and I-set initialized as empty (lines 3–9). In the next phase (lines 10–20), the nodes are dequeued one at a time, with the I-sets and D-sets (for t) updated according to the mechanism described in Fig. 2.6.

We illustrate the steps of Algorithm 3 using an example. The input DAG is given in Fig. 2.7 (top left), and there is a redundant edge (colored in red) that FEDRR is supposed to detect. The algorithm starts with setting initial values for the D-set and the I-set and enqueuing those node with no incoming edges, as shown on the top right of Fig. 2.7. The result is shown on the bottom right of Fig. 2.7.

The algorithm starts with setting initial values for the D-set and the I-set and enqueuing those node with no incoming edges, as shown on the top of Fig. 2.7 on the right. For this sample DAG, the result is shown on the bottom right of Fig. 2.7.

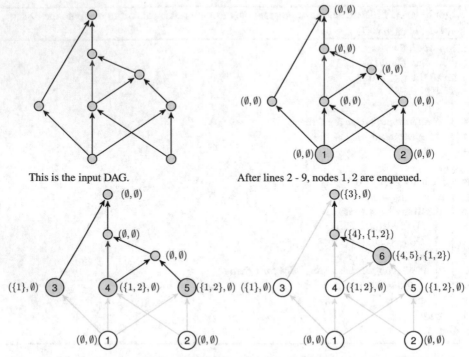

This is the input DAG.

After lines 2 - 9, nodes 1, 2 are enqueued.

Nodes 1, 2 dequeued, D−set and I−set updated on 3, 4, 5. Nodes 3, 4, 5 enqueued.

After nodes 3, 4, 5 dequeued, D-set and I-set updated on nodes 6, 7, 8 (7, 8 not enqueued yet, thus not numbered). Node 6 enqueued.

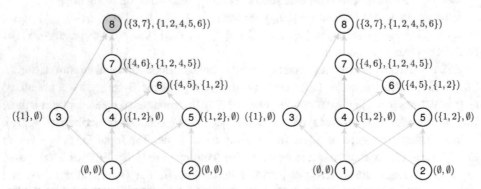

Node 6 dequeued, D-set and I-set updated on node 7. Node 7 enqueued. Node 7 dequeued, D-set and I-set updated on node 8. Node 8 enqueued.

Node 8 dequeued, queue is empty.

Fig. 2.7 Example illustrating step-through run of Algorithm 3

Correctness

The correctness of the algorithm can be proved using mathematical induction by showing $I[v_i] = I_{v_i}$ and $D[v_i] = D_{v_i}$ after node v_i is dequeued (line 11) for $i = 1 \ldots |V|$.

Proof $i = 1$. The first dequeued node must be a node with no incoming edges. This means $I_{v_1} = \emptyset$ and $D_{v_1} = \emptyset$. As both $I[v_1] = \emptyset$ and $D[v_1] = \emptyset$ from lines 4 and 5, we have $I[v_1] = I_{v_1}$ and $D[v_1] = D_{v_1}$.

Suppose $I[v_i] = I_{v_i}$ and $D[v_i] = D_{v_i}$ is true for $i = 1 \ldots k - 1$. For $i = k$, then we have $D[v_k] = \{v \mid (v, v_k) \in E\}$ and $I[v_k] = \bigcup_j (D[v_{k_j}] \cup I[v_{k_j}])$, where $v_{k_j} \in \{v \mid (v, v_k) \in E\}$. Based on the definition of D_v, we have $D_{v_k} = \{v \mid (v, v_k) \in E\} = D[v_k]$. From the induction hypothesis, we have $I[v_i] = I_{v_i}$ and $D[v_i] = D_{v_i}$ for $i = 1 \ldots k - 1$. This means $I[v_k] = \bigcup_j (D[v_{k_j}] \cup I[v_{k_j}]) = \bigcup_j (D_{v_{k_j}} \cup I_{v_{k_j}}) = I_{v_k}$. $\square$

Time Complexity Analysis

The topological sorting itself takes $O(|V| + |E|)$ time [47]. With the computation of D-set and I-set, the total time is $O(\sum_{(u,v) \in E}(|D_v| + |I_v|) + |V| + |E|)$. When $|E| = O(|V|)$ (which is the case for both SNOMED CT and GO), the running time is $O(\sum_v(|D_v| + |I_v|) + |V| + |E|)$. If we let $c = \frac{\sum_v(|D_v| + |I_v|)}{|V|}$, then the running time is in $O(c \cdot |V| + |E|)$. Based on the definition of D_v and I_v, $\sum_v(|D_v| + |I_v|)$ is the size of transitive closure pairs shown in Tables 2.3 and 2.4. Even though the worst-case running time is $O(|V|^2)$(when $c = |V|$), c is a relatively small constant for ontological systems in practice. This is validated by our experimental results shown in Tables 2.3 and 2.4. For the 2015-03-01 version of SNOMED CT, $c = \frac{5,408,010}{315,904} = 17.12$, and for the 2015-05-01 version of GO, $c = \frac{557,550}{42,979} = 12.97$.

2.2.2 Experiments Performed and the Results Obtained for SNOMED CT, Gene Ontology, and the UMLS

The following subsections briefly discuss the results obtained. For detailed results, analysis, and discussions, please see [48].

Experimental Environment

To detect redundant *is-a* relations from SNOMED CT and Gene Ontology, we ran the FEDRR method on a MacBook Pro running the Mac OS X Yosemite with 16 GB RAM and Intel Core i7 processor. FEDRR was implemented in Java programming language based on JDK7.

Redundant is-a Relations in SNOMED CT

We ran the FEDRR method on 5 versions of SNOMED CT (U.S. edition) from 2013 to 2015 dated on 2013-09-01, 2014-03-01, 2014-09-01, 2015-03-01, and 2015-09-01. Table 2.3 summarizes the result of each version including numbers of concepts, *is-a* relations, and transitive closure pairs (TC), and number of redundant *is-a* relations (RR); percentage of redundant

Table 2.4 Summary of the results for 10 versions of Gene Ontology. TC: number of transitive closure pairs, RR: number of redundant *is-a* relations, RR%: percentage of redundant *is-a* relations among transitive closure pairs, T (ms): time taken in milliseconds

Version	# Concepts	# *is-a* Relations	TC	RR	RR%	T (ms)
2014-08-01	41,436	66,544	517,092	497	0.0961	1,372
2014-09-01	41,694	66,995	522,741	502	0.0960	1,472
2014-10-01	41,867	67,536	528,821	631	0.1193	1,455
2014-11-01	42,012	69,300	541,718	1,031	0.1903	1,497
2014-12-01	42,189	69,887	545,168	1,193	0.2188	1,425
2015-01-01	42,329	70,272	544,210	1,277	0.2347	1,510
2015-02-01	42,466	70,724	546,158	1,420	0.2600	1,549
2015-03-01	42,588	71,032	548,006	1,463	0.2670	1,542
2015-04-01	42,805	71,549	552,367	1,552	0.2810	1,437
2015-05-01	42,979	71,954	557,550	1,609	0.2886	1,538

is-a relations (RR%) among transitive closure pairs; and computing time in milliseconds to detect redundant *is-a* relations. For example, for the 2015-09-01 version, there were 320,911 concepts, 476,226 *is-a* relations, 5,511,334 transitive closure pairs, and 372 redundant *is-a* relations; the percentage of the redundant *is-a* relations among the transitive closure pairs is 0.00675%; and it took about 16 s to complete. For each version, it only took a few seconds to identify all the redundant *is-a* relations, indicating the efficiency of FEDRR.

Redundant is-a Relations in Gene Ontology
We ran the FEDRR method to detect redundant *is-a* relations in 10 versions of Gene Ontology from 2014-08-01 to 2015-05-01 updated monthly. Table 2.4 summarizes the basic results of each version. For instance, for the 2015-05-01 version, there were 42,979 concepts, 71,954 *is-a* relations, 557,550 transitive closure pairs, and 1,609 redundant *is-a* relations; the percentage of the redundant *is-a* relations among the transitive closure pairs is 0.2886%; and it took 1,538 ms to complete. As the number of concepts and *is-a* relations were increasing, the number and percentage of redundant *is-a* relations (RR) were monotonically increasing every month and increased more than twice from the 2014-08-01 version (497; 0.0961%) to the 2015-05-01 version (1,609; 0.2886%). For each version, it only took a couple of seconds to identify all the redundant *is-a* relations, indicating the efficiency of FEDRR.

Redundant is-a Relations in UMLS
We ran the FEDRR method to detect redundant *is-a* relations from over 190 source vocabularies integrated in the UMLS (2015AB release). Since the original occurrences of concept names are preserved and identified as AUIs in the UMLS, we used AUIs and relations

Table 2.5 Summary of the results for source vocabularies in UMLS (2015AB release) with redundant relations. AUI: Atom Unique Identifier, TC: number of transitive closure pairs, RR: number of redundant *is-a* relations, T (ms): time taken in milliseconds

Version	# AUIs	# *is-a* Relations	TC	RR	RR%	T (ms)
SNOMEDCT_US	846,444	476,055	5,511,334	372	0.00675	28,977
SNOMEDCT_VET	85,939	19,832	29,688	7	0.024	954
GO	148,900	71,687	554,859	1,576	0.2840	9,128
NCI	270,618	119,707	701,986	20	0.0028	5,881
HPO	18,175	14,762	117,366	101	0.0861	502
UMD	34,124	10,750	37,732	20	0.0530	1,906

between AUIs to detect redundant *is-a* relations. We also filtered out inactive *is-a* relations in the UMLS before applying the FEDRR method.

Based on our experiment, the concept graph in terms of AUI is acyclic, and FEDRR completes the exhaustive search for all the sources in our experiments. Six sources were found to have redundant *is-a* relations (see Table 2.5): SNOMEDCT_US (2015_09_01), SNOMEDCT_VET (2015_04_01), GO (2015_04_04), NCI (1502D), HPO (2015_04_20), and UMD (2015AA). For instance, in HPO, there were 18,175 AUIs, 14,762 *is-a* relations, 117,366 transitive closure pairs, and 101 redundant *is-a* relations. Moreover, it took FEDRR less than 30 s to detect redundant *is-a* relations for each of these source vocabularies.

Evaluation

Even though in most cases redundant edges should be removed, in some cases the redundancy is caused by a mistake of an edge along the indirect path. For example, in Fig. 2.8, the assertion that "*Bilateral congenital dislocation of hip*" *is-a* "*Congenital dislocation of right hip*" is most likely in error. This is because a concept involving "bilateral" should not be a subclass of a concept of limited laterality: "right" (but not "left"). Removing this edge would have automatically eliminated the redundancy of the detected relation.

To evaluate the performance of FEDRR's detection of redundant *is-a* relations from original sources of SNOMED CT and GO, a random sample of 30 redundant relations from SNOMED CT (2015-03-01 version) and 50 from GO (2015-05-01 version) were selected and manually reviewed by two human annotators. One annotator was asked to manually verify if the redundant hierarchical relations identified by FEDRR are correct.

The other annotator was asked to review each redundant relation and provide on feedback if the redundant relation (direct edge) should be removed or an edge in the indirect path should be removed. For instance, Fig. 2.9 presents an example of redundant relation from GO manually reviewed by the second annotator. In this case, the annotator's feedback is to

Fig. 2.8 A visualized example
of redundant *is-a* relation in
SNOMED CT

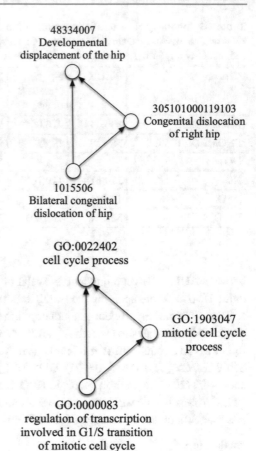

48334007
Developmental
displacement of the hip

305101000119103
Congenital dislocation
of right hip

1015506
Bilateral congenital
dislocation of hip

Fig. 2.9 A visualized example
of redundant *is-a* relation in
GO

GO:0022402
cell cycle process

GO:1903047
mitotic cell cycle
process

GO:0000083
regulation of transcription
involved in G1/S transition
of mitotic cell cycle

remove the direct edge. For cases like the one shown in Fig. 2.8, the annotator's feedback is
to remove the indirect edge that is incorrect.

The first annotator verified that all of the redundant *is-a* relations identified by FEDRR
are correct, that is, 100% accuracy. Based on the second annotators evaluation, it was seen
that among 30 redundant *is-a* relations in SNOMED CT, 24 (80%) should have direct edge
removed, and 6 (20%) should have indirect edge removed. Among 50 redundant *is-a* relations
in GO, 45 (90%) should have direct edge removed, and 5 (10%) should have indirect edge
removed.

To evaluate the performance of FEDRR's detection of redundant hierarchical relations
from UMLS, a random sample of 30 redundant relations detected from the SNOMEDCT_US
in the UMLS was selected and manually reviewed by the first annotator. The annotator
verified that all the 30 redundant relations identified by FEDRR are correct (100% accuracy).

2.2.3   Further Discussions of the Findings

Comparison with Related Work

There has been related work on exploring redundant relations in biomedical ontologies or terminologies [49–53]. Bodenreider [49] investigated the redundancy of hierarchical relations across biomedical terminologies in the UMLS. Different from Bodenreider's work, FEDRR focuses on developing a fast and scalable approach to detect redundant hierarchical relations within a single ontology.

Gu et al. [50] investigated five categories of possibly incorrect relationship assignment including redundant relations in FMA. The redundant relations were detected based on the interplay between the *is-a* and other structural relationships (*part-of*, *tributary-of*, *branch-of*). A review of 20 samples from possible redundant *part-of* relations validated 14 errors, a 70% correctness. FEDRR differs from this work in two ways. Firstly, FEDRR aims to provide an efficient algorithm to identify redundant hierarchical relations from large ontologies with 100% accuracy. Secondly, FEDRR can be used for detecting redundant relations in all DAGs with the transitivity property.

Mougin [51] studied redundant relations as well as missing relations in GO. The identification of redundant relations was based on the combination of relationships including *is-a* and *is-a*, *is-a* and *part-of*, *part-of* and *part-of*, and *is-a* and *positively-regulates*. FEDRR's main focus is to provide a generalizable and efficient approach to detecting redundant hierarchical relations in any ontology, which has been illustrated by applying it to all the UMLS source vocabularies. Moreover, the redundant hierarchical relations detected by FEDRR were evaluated by human experts, while only a number of redundant relations was reported in [51] without human annotator's validation.

Bodenreider [54], Mougin and Bodenreider [55], and Halper et al. [56] studied various approaches to removing cyclic hierarchical relations in the UMLS. Although no cycles have been detected in the current UMLS in terms of the AUI, such approaches [54–56] to detecting and removing cyclic relations are needed before FEDRR can be applied. This is because FEDRR is based on the topological sorting of a graph, which requires no cycles in a graph.

Conclusion: Detecting and removing redundant relations is an important quality improvement task for biomedical ontologies because non-redundancy is the basic premise of all semantic measures derived from ontological structures, such as semantic distance between concepts and ontology mapping and alignment. We introduced FEDRR for fast and exhaustive detection of redundant hierarchical relations in ontological hierarchies. Our algorithm runs in linear time to the size of the ontological structure in practice.

Using FEDRR, we performed a systematic and exhaustive search of redundant *is-a* relations in two large ontological systems in biomedicine: SNOMED CT and Gene Ontology, as well as all the source vocabularies in the UMLS. The algorithmic core of FEDRR is easy to implement and extremely efficient. In our extensive experiments on real-world, large ontological structures, it took less than 20 s for FEDRR to process SNOMED CT and Gene Ontology. Moreover, FEDRR is a general approach and can be applied to detect redundant relations in other hierarchical structures.

2.3   Cross-Ontology Examination

Most existing works have focused on developing auditing methods utilizing the knowledge (e.g., terms, relationships) provided within a targeted ontology. This section proposes a novel cross-ontology method, Cross-Ontology Hierarchical Relationship Examination (COHeRE), to detect possible errors and inconsistencies in hierarchical relationships across multiple biomedical ontologies in the UMLS [2]. COHeRE leverages the MapReduce cloud computing technique for systematic, large-scale ontology quality assurance work. Inconsistencies uncovered using COHeRE involve UMLS concept pairs related by different types of relationships in disparate source vocabularies. For example, *"Prolonged depressive adjustment reaction"* is related to *"Adjustment disorder with depressed mood"* through the *is-a* relationship in SNOMED CT, while *"Prolonged depressive reaction"* is related to *"Adjustment disorder with depressed mood"* through the *sibling* relationship in ICD9CM (Fig. 2.10). Since not all such relations can be correct the inconsistencies provide immediate candidates for auditing and change. For example, the *sibling* relationship in Fig. 2.10 should probably be changed to *is-a*, in ICD9CM.

2.3.1   Steps to Detect Hierarchical Inconsistencies

Figure 2.11 shows the overview of the proposed pipeline of steps for COHeRE. First, the UMLS concepts and relations are taken as the input; relations are filtered according to certain criteria; and relations claimed in source vocabularies are aggregated for each concept pair. Second, inconsistent relations are detected if a concept pair has disparate relations in different

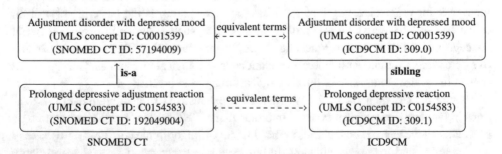

Fig. 2.10 Example of inconsistent relations in SNOMED CT and ICD9CM integrated in the UMLS

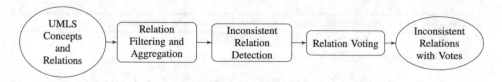

Fig. 2.11 Overview of the proposed method COHeRE

source vocabularies. Finally, the inconsistent relations are voted by source vocabularies, and the voting result together with the inconsistent relations are the output.

Relation Filtering and Aggregation

Material Preparation The MRCONSO (1.41GB) and MRREL (5.48GB) distribution files in the UMLS 2014AB release are used as the input for concepts and relations between concepts, respectively. Since UMLS is multilingual and covers a wide range of vocabularies, a subset of most relevant source vocabularies are manually selected to perform the cross-ontology examination for this study. Hence terms that are not in the subset of source vocabularies are discarded from MRCONSO. In addition, concepts with terms containing word *unspecified* or *NOS* (Not Otherwise Specified) are filtered out from MRCONSO, since such terms are very likely to cause error-prone relations in the integrated MRREL.

Relation Filtering Each relation record in MRREL can be represented as (C_1, C_2, R, RA, S), where C_1 and C_2 form a concept pair, R is the relationship between C_1 and C_2 indicating C_2 R C_1, RA is the relationship attribute of R, and S is the source vocabulary. Since every source relationship is represented in two directions in separate rows in UMLS, analyzing both directions of a concept pair is redundant. For example, if a concept pair (C_1, C_2) is related through the *CHD* relationship with the *is-a* relationship attribute, then (C_2, C_1) is symmetrically related through the *PAR* relationship with the *inverse is-a* relation attribute. To avoid duplicated analysis, only one direction *CHD* is used for analyzing this concept pair. Generally, concept pairs with relationship *CHD, RN, SIB, SY, AQ* or *RO* are used for the cross-ontology analysis. In addition, a concept pair is discarded if the concepts share the same unique identifier *CUI*, since COHeRE will only investigate relationships between distinct concepts. Concept pairs with relationship attribute RA as *mapped from* or *mapped to* are also ignored, since they are generated by UMLS and represent mappings between source vocabularies. Due to the large size of the MREEL file, this filtering process is implemented using MapReduce (Mapper in Algorithm 4) to enable parallel computing.

Relation Aggregation For each concept pair (C_1, C_2), source relationships are aggregated into the format of

$$(C_1, C_2) \rightarrow (R_1, RA_1, S_1) \mid (R_2, RA_2, S_2) \mid \ldots \mid (R_n, RA_n, S_n).$$

Since COHeRE aims to audit ontologies utilizing external knowledge, (C_1, C_2) are discarded if they are multiply related in a single source vocabulary, that is, there exist i and j such

---

Algorithm 4: MapReduce algorithm for Relation Filtering and Aggregation.

---

1 **Input:** Relations in MRREL $\{(C_1, C_2, R, RA, S)\}$
2 **Output:** Aggregated relations by concept pairs:

$$\{(C_1, C_2) \rightarrow (R_1, RA_1, S_1)|(R_2, RA_2, S_2)|\ldots|(R_n, RA_n, S_n)\}$$

3 **class** MAPPER
4 Setup a HashSet H and load it with all the relevant concepts in MRCONSO using
  DistributedCache.
5 **method** MAP((C_1, C_2, R, RA, S))
6 **if** H *contains both* C_1 *and* C_2, C_1 *and* C_2 *are not identical,* R *is not in* {CHD, RN, SIB, SY,
  AQ, RO}, *and* RA *is* mapped from *or* mapped to **then**
7 | EMIT($(C_1, C_2), (R, RA, S)$)
8 **end**

9 **class** REDUCER
10 **method** REDUCE($(C_1, C_2), \{(R_1, RA_1, S_1), (R_2, RA_2, S_2), \ldots, (R_n, RA_n, S_n)\}$)
11 Setup a HashMap M for source vocabularies and relationships.
12 **if** C_1 *and* C_2 *are not multiply related for each source vocabulary in* M **then**
13 | EMIT($(C_1, C_2), \{(R_1, RA_1, S_1)|(R_2, RA_2, S_2)|\ldots|(R_n, RA_n, S_n)\}$)
14 **end**

---

that $R_i \neq R_j$ but $S_i = S_j$. For example, in the source vocabulary *SNOMEDCT_US*, concepts "*Acetaminophen*" (C0000970) and "*Acetaminophen 160mg/5mL elixir*" (C0973757) are related through two relationships: *CHD (is-a)* and *RO (has active ingredient)*. Such inconsistencies are discarded at the single source level. The relation aggregation process is implemented as a MapReduce Reducer in Algorithm 4.

In sum, concept pair (C_1, C_2) with relationship R and relationship attribute RA is filtered out if one of the following criteria is met:

- the relationship R is not *CHD, RN, SIB, SY, AQ* or *RO*;
- the two concepts C_1 and C_2 share the same unique identifier *CUI*;
- the relation attribute RA is *mapped from* or *mapped to*;
- if the two concepts C_1 and C_2 are multiply related in a single source vocabulary after relation aggregation.

Inconsistent Relation Detection

For each pair of concepts obtained in the Relation Filtering and Aggregation step, the concepts are related either in a single source vocabulary or in multiple source vocabularies. For instance, the concepts "*Arginine supplement*" (C3853287) and "*Arginine and glutamine supplement*" (C3853286) are related through *CHD* only in a single source vocabulary *SNOMEDCT_US* (No. 1 in Table 2.6); the concepts "*Hexosamines*" (C0019478) and "*Fructosamine*" (C0060765) are related through *CHD* in both *MSH* and *NDFRT* (No. 2 in

Table 2.6 Examples of concept pairs after the Relation Filtering and Aggregation process

No.	Concept pair (C_1, C_2)	Relationships and source vocabularies $\{(R, RA, S)\}$
1	*Arginine supplement (C3853287), Arginine and glutamine supplement (C3853286)*	*CHD, is a, SNOMEDCT_US*
2	*Hexosamines (C0019478) Fructosamine (C0060765)*	*CHD, null, MSH	CHD, null, NDFRT*
3	*17-Oxosteroid (C0000167), Androstenedione (C0002860)*	*SIB, null, CPM	CHD, null, MSH	CHD, null, NDFRT*

Table 2.6); the concepts "*17-Oxosteroid*" (C0000167) and "*Androstenedione*" (C0002860) are related through *SIB* in *CPM* and *CHD* in both *MSH* and *NDFRT* (No. 3 in Table 2.6).

Concepts pairs related in a single vocabulary are considered consistent (see the decision tree in Fig. 2.12). For each concept pair with multiple source vocabularies, the concepts are either related through homogeneous relationships (e.g., No. 2 in Table 2.6) or non-homogeneous relationships (e.g., No. 3 in Table 2.6). Concept pairs related through homogeneous relationships are considered consistent, while those related through non-homogeneous relationships are considered inconsistent and collected to facilitate further analysis.

Relation Voting

The inconsistent concept pairs detected above have non-homogeneous relationships across different source vocabularies. A voting module is developed to rank the non-homogeneous relationships by the number of claimed source vocabularies. If the relationship with the most votes has at least 2 votes, then it will serve as a suggestion for correcting potential errors in the inconsistent source vocabularies; otherwise, no suggestion will be made by COHeRE. Take row 3 in Table 2.6 as an example, the *CHD* relationship receives 2 votes from the source vocabularies *MSH* and *NDFRT*, and the *SIB* relationship receives 1 vote from the source vocabulary *CPM*. Hence *CHD* relationship could be suggested to correct potential error or inconsistency in the source vocabulary *CPM*. The output of COHeRE are the inconsistent concept pairs and suggested relationships with the most votes.

Fig. 2.12 Decision tree for inconsistent relation detection using the example concept pairs provided in Table 2.6 as the input. The numbers in the curly brackets indicate the row numbers in Table 2.6

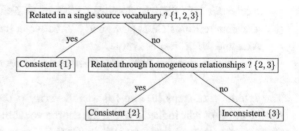

2.3.2   Inconsistencies Uncovered and Evaluation Performed

The following summarizes the results obtained. For detailed explanations and analysis, please see [57].

After the Relation Filtering and Aggregation step, 11,921,502 distinct concept pairs were obtained. Among these, 11,372,069 pairs were related in a single source vocabulary, and 549,433 pairs were related in multiple source vocabularies. After the Inconsistent Relation Detection step, 138,987 concept pairs were found with inconsistent relationships across multiple source vocabularies.

Evaluation

Since hierarchical relationships are dominant in biomedical ontologies, this study focused on evaluating two types of inconsistent relationships [*CHD, RO*] and [*CHD, SIB*]. A random sample of 40 UMLS concept pairs with inconsistent relationships (20 for each type) was selected and manually reviewed by a human expert.

For each given pair of UMLS concepts, the expert was required to perform the following procedures:

(a) Check if there are terms mapping to them in each source vocabulary involved, and keep records of identifier codes for each term identified in a source vocabulary.
(b) For each relationship between the two concepts, check if the relationship is indeed claimed in the corresponding source vocabulary.
(c) For the relationship with the highest votes as at least 2, choose "agree," "disagree," or "not sure" to rate if the expert agrees that it can be used as the correct relationship for the concept pair to resolve inconsistency. For the case that there is 1 vote for each relationship involved, specify one relationship as the correct relationship or answer "not sure."

Take as an example the UMLS concepts "*Osteosarcoma metastatic*" (C0278512) and "*Extraskeletal osteosarcoma metastatic*" (C0855050) related through *CHD (is-a)* in *NCI* and *SIB* in *MDR*:

(a) Terms mapping to the concept "*Osteosarcoma metastatic*" (C0278512) include *C7781* in *NCI* and *10031246* in *MDR*. And terms mapping to "*Extraskeletal osteosarcoma metastatic*" (C0855050) include *C8808* in *NCI* and *10015849* in *MDR*.
(b) The relationships *CHD (is-a)* and *SIB* between the two concepts are indeed claimed in *NCI* and *MDR*, respectively.
(c) The expert specifies that *CHD (is-a)* is the correct relationship.

The intention of steps (a) and (b) was to verify if the detected inconsistent relationships for the concept pair indeed exist in the source vocabularies or are caused by the integration process of source vocabularies into the UMLS. They are essential for evaluating COHeRE's ability to filter out noisy information the integration of UMLS may cause and detect valid inconsistent relationships across different ontologies.

It was verified that all the 40 concept pairs have mapping terms in the involved source vocabularies. For a total of 95 individual relations (note that one concept pair have multiple individual relations in different source vocabularies), only 4 of them were found not claimed in the corresponding source vocabulary. For instance, the *is-a* relation between "*Metformin*" (C0025598) and "*Metformin hydrochloride 1000 MG Oral Tablet*" (C0978482) was no longer active in *SNOMEDCT_US*, but still included in the UMLS. In general, 95.8% (91/95) of the individual relations detected by COHeRE are valid.

For cases where the relationship with highest votes is at least 2, there were 19 concept pairs, among which 14 (73.7%) concept pairs were agreed by the expert, 2 disagreed, and 3 not sure. For the case that there is 1 vote for each relationship involved, there were 21 concept pairs, among which, 19 concept pairs were specified a correct relationship by the expert, and 2 not sure.

Manual examination of the verified result indicates the following facts:

- *ICD9CM, MSH,* and MDR sometimes classify concepts related through *CHD* as *SIB*. "*Dermatitis Herpetiformis*" (C0011608) and "*Juvenile dermatitis herpetiformis*" (C0152092) are related through *CHD (is-a)* in *SNOMEDCT_US*, and *SIB* in *ICD9CM*; "*Neurites*" (C0085103) and "*Axon*" (C0004461) are related through *CHD* in *GO* and FMA, and *SIB* in *MSH*; "*Ventricular Dysfunction*" (C0242973) and "*Right Ventricular Dysfunctions*" (C0242707) are related through *CHD* in *MSH, NCI, NDFRT,* and *SIB* in *MDR*.

- *SNOMED_CT* and *NDFRT* show inconsistencies regarding to relations between pharmacologic substances and clinical drugs. For instance, the pharmacologic substance "*Buprenorphine/Naloxone*" (C1169989) and the clinical drug "*Buprenorphine 8 MG / Naloxone 2 MG Sublingual Tablet*" (C1168831) are related through *CHD* in *SNOMED_CT* and *NDFRT*, and *RO (has ingredient)* in *RXNORM* and *VANDF*. However, the pharmacologic substance "*Potassium Chloride*" (C0032825) and the clinical drug "*Potassium Chloride 1 MEQ/ML Oral Solution*" (C0979640) are indeed related through *RO (has active ingredient)* in *SNOMED_CT*, and through *RO (has ingredient)* in *NDFRT*. This indicates that *SNOMED_US* and *NDFRT* are inconsistent for relating clinical drugs with pharmacologic substances.

- *SNOMED_CT* sometimes relates body parts using *CHD (is-a)* instead of *part-of*. For instance, "*Fifth lumbar vertebra*" (C0223552) and "*Arch of fifth lumbar vertebra*" (C0223553) are related through *CHD* in *SNOMEDCT_US*, and *RO (regional part of)* in *FMA*.

2.3.3   Further Findings of the Work

Distinction from Related Work

COHeRE leverages the knowledge across different ontologies to detect possible errors, which is distinct from most existing ontology quality assurance approaches utilizing the knowledge provided within a targeted ontology such as the ones discussed in Sects. 2.1 and 4.1. COHeRE also differs from the approach discussed in Sect. 5.1, where the structural disparity between SNOMED CT's Body Structure sub-hierarchy and FMA was investigated using a cross-ontology method, but the scope was limited to ontological terms relating to human body structure. In [52], Mougin and Grabar exhaustively studied multiply-related concepts within the UMLS, and explored why the multiply-related concepts occur and whether they are inherited from source vocabularies or introduced by the UMLS integration. It was reported that a quarter of multiply-related concepts in UMLS are inherited from source vocabularies [52]. COHeRE differs from [52] in two ways. One is that COHeRE adopts only a subset of source vocabularies that are most relevant for cross-ontology examination. The other is that COHeRE aims to achieve an effective filtering mechanism to remove the multiply-related concepts caused by the UMLS integration, and utilize the actual inconsistent relationships across multiple source vocabularies to detect inconsistencies and facilitate ontology quality assurance.

Conceptualization Difference Analysis

Manual analysis showed conceptual difference between ontologies. Take the concept pair "*Nipple neoplasm*" (C1112166) and "*Benign nipple neoplasm*" (C1332519) as an example, COHeRE detected two inconsistent relationships: *CHD (is-a)* in the source vocabulary *NCI*, and *SIB* in the source vocabulary *MDR*. In *NCI*, "*Nipple neoplasm*" is classified into "*Benign nipple neoplasm*" and "*Malignant nipple neoplasm*." In *MDR*, "neoplasm" is classified according to "benign," "malignant," and "unspecified." "*Nipple neoplasm*" is classified under "*Breast neoplasms unspecified malignancy*," and "*Benign nipple neoplasm*" is classified under "*Breast neoplasms benign*." Hence the detected inconsistency is due to the conceptual difference. Although concept terms containing "unspecified" were filtered out by COHeRE, other terms classified under such terms were still included for the inconsistency detection (e.g., "*Nipple neoplasm*" under "*Breast neoplasms unspecified malignancy*"). To avoid this, the hierarchical information provided by UMLS (the distribution file *MRHIER*) can be used to remove the descendant terms of those terms containing "unspecified."

Limitations

First, this study relies on the UMLS knowledge source, and it is not generalizable to domains lacking an integrated ontological system. Second, this study is limited in the number of concept pairs with inconsistent relationships evaluated. Third, this study only focused on evaluating two types of inconsistent relationships ([*CHD, SIB*] and [*CHD, RO*]). Evaluating more types of concept pairs may reveal more interesting inconsistencies. Fourth, this study did not investigate concept pairs that are multiply related in a single source vocabulary. It would be interesting to study inconsistent relationships occurring in a single source vocabulary. Lastly, if the ontologies integrated in UMLS are given in the Web Ontology Language (OWL) and the relations are defined as mutually exclusive, then simple OWL inferencing should be able to detect these inconsistencies.

Conclusion: This section presented a novel cross-ontology method, COHeRE, to detect possible errors and inconsistencies in hierarchical relationships across multiple biomedical ontologies. COHeRE leverages the UMLS knowledge source and the MapReduce cloud computing technique for systematic, large-scale ontology quality assurance work. COHeRE is effective in detecting inconsistent hierarchical relations among UMLS source ontologies for quality assurance. The effectiveness of COHeRE indicates that UMLS provides a promising environment to enhance qualities of biomedical ontologies.

2.4   Multi-type Relations

In this section, we introduce a novel method for Ontology Quality Assurance by exploiting the interaction of multiple types of relationships, called *Motif Checking* (MOCH).

MOCH has a unique combination of features. It leverages antonyms to uncover the disjointness relation between concepts, not explicitly modeled in FMA; It combines the interaction of multiple times of relationships in the context of the disjointness property to achieve greater auditing specificity; It is computationally scalable, through the use of Semantic Web technology, so small graph motifs can be exhaustively enumerated and systematically checked; It has a strong rule-based flavor and is generally applicable to other ontological systems (not just FMA). The primary use case considered in this section is FMA [58], which involves five main relational subtypes: *subclass (is-a), part-of, regional-part-of, constitutional-part-of, and systemic-part-of.* Such subtypes are explicitly supported by the Foundational Model Explorer (http://fme.biostr.washington.edu:8080).

The standard semantics for *part-of* is this following: class A is classified as *part-of* class B if every instance of A has some instance of B as a part. This can be formally expressed in description logic [59] as: A $part - of$ B if and only if $A \sqsubseteq \exists p B$, where p is the relation capturing the *part-of* relation at the instance level. By chaining of logical implications (i.e., $X \sqsubseteq Y$ and $Y \sqsubseteq Z$ implies $X \sqsubseteq Z$), we obtain the following as a general principle, which we call *subclass-partonomy mixing (Fig. 2.13): if A is-a B, and B is part-of C, then A is part-of C.*

Does FMA conform to this? To answer this question, consider an example

$A = Male$ *urinary system* (FMA222947),
$B = Urinary$ *system* (FMA7159), and
$C = Female$ *human body* (FMA67812).

about which FMA asserted two relational instances:

Fig. 2.13 The subclass-partonomy mixing motif. Dotted line represents the inferred relation instance. This principle is sometimes called "relation dependence [26]"

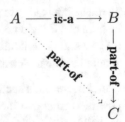

1. *Male urinary system* (*A*) is a subclass of *Urinary system* (*B*), and
2. *Urinary system* (*B*) is a part of *Female human body* (*C*).

Therefore, we obtain "*Male urinary system*" is a *part-of* "*Female human body*," implying that the two classes should share instances, which is of course incorrect because "*Male urinary system*" and "*Female human body*" are disjoint classes. We know this based on *external* knowledge about canonical human anatomy, which is not represented in FMA. Therefore, such errors cannot be detected by checking logical consistency of FMA because it is under-specified with respect to disjointness.

The main objective of MOCH is to provide an exhaustive, computationally scalable approach to analyze the effect of interactions of multiple types of relations in ontological systems and provide a unique source of information valuable for quality assurance. This unique feature comes from the idea of "negative thinking:" motifs are designed to capture seemingly impossible configurations, aided by syntactic grounding on possible disjointness of concepts using antonyms in the names.

MOCH represents patterns of such interactions as small labeled sub-graph motifs, whose nodes represent class variables, and labeled edges represent the type of relationship. The motifs can be designed in such a way to deliberately capture "impossible" or "inconsistent" situations, such as the one on top of Fig. 2.14. If an actual subgraph is found which matches this motif, such as that shown in the lower part of Fig. 2.14, then it represents an auditing candidate. It invites us to re-examine the two asserted relational instances, "*Male urinary system*" is a subclass of "*Urinary system*," and "*Urinary system*" is a part of "*Female human body*," one of which is likely to be incorrect. In this particular example, the latter is incorrect because not all Urinary systems (male and female) are a part of Female human body.

For the purpose of this work, since we are not working with direct sibling classes, we use implied disjointness property between classes using lexical information in class names. That is, we leverage *antonyms* for likely (but not always) disjointness, where disjointness of classes A and B means that no instance is both A as well as B; in set notation, $A \cap B = \emptyset$. For example, we infer that "*Male urinary system*" and "*Female human body*" are disjoint classes because their use of the antonym pair (male, female). (And indeed these are disjoint classes because an instance of "*Male urinary system*" cannot be also an instance of "*Female human body*").

We selected anatomically relevant antonym-pairs from a total of 400 common antonyms for this work.

Fig. 2.14 A disjoint open jaw
motif (above) and a matching
instance in FMA (below;
numbers displayed are FMA
ID)

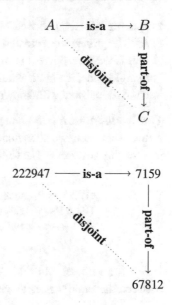

Note that classes using antonyms are not automatically disjoint. For example, it likely
takes a domain expert to conclude that the class "*Transitional myocyte of right branch of
atrioventricular bundle*" (FMA263172), containing the substring "right," is disjoint from
"*Region of wall of left ventricle*" (FMA85471) which contains the substring "left." The
heuristics we exploit is that in some cases, especially gender, such classes are indeed disjoint.
Nonetheless, some gender specific information may not be explicitly reflected in class names,
such as "*Prostate*" (FMA9600), a male only anatomical class which does not contain "male"
in the label.

2.4.1   Steps of the Motif Checking Approach

The MOCH approach for identifying FMA auditing fragments for review involves the following steps: (1) acquiring FMA data and generating RDF data store; (2) creating SPARQL
queries to encode two-node, three-node motifs; (3) executing the motifs to obtain detected
configurations [60].

Acquiring FMA Data
The model underlying the FMA is a frame-based representation with 78,977 concepts including macroscopic, microscopic, and sub-cellular canonical anatomy. For our analysis, we used
the legacy version of the OWL translation of FMA from the Open Biomedical Ontology
(OBO) Foundry. The FMA OWL version from OBO foundry is distributed as an RDF/XML-
based serialization that enables it to be stored in a RDF data store and made available to be
queried via SPARQL over internet protocol.

Preparing SPARQL-Based Motif Templates

SPARQL queries were created in three distinct categories corresponding to the three types of motifs we investigated: two-node motifs, three-node motifs, and arbitrary-length motifs. For single node, the motif would amount to checking cycles, which we have not found any in FMA, consistent with known-observations [59].

Two-Node Motif A two-node motif is the smallest motif of interest. With one relationship instance between two class nodes, this become the basic building block of primitive asserted relationship instances. The following motifs are considered:

> (I) *A is-a B*, and also *A* is a *part-of B* at the same time;
> (II) *A is-a B*, and *A* and *B* involve antonyms in their class names;
> (III) *A* is a *part-of B*, and *A* and *B* involve antonyms in their class names.

We were interested in this kind of motifs because such multiple types of relationships between the same classes looked counterintuitive at first.

Three-Node Motif With a single edge relation linking three node classes, we considered 12 motifs as displayed in Table 2.7.

Principal Ideal Exploration One of the limitations of three-node motifs is that the classes at the two ends are separated by precisely two links, i.e., two asserted relationship instances. We use Principal Ideal Explorer (PIE) to extend MOCH to account for situations where classes at the two ends are separated by *an arbitrary number of links*, exploiting the transitivity property of *is-a* and *part-of*. Thus PIE extends motif analysis to principal ideals to achieve completeness of quality checking throughout the hierarchy.

The idea behind PIE is that properties that hold for more general ("ancestor") classes in taxonomies and partonomies also hold for more specific ("descendant") classes. If class *A* and class *B* are connected by a sequence of relational instances (*is-a* or *part-of*), *in the same direction*, then *A* and *B* should not be disjoint (otherwise it is not possible to inherit properties from the ancestor class). For an illustration, Fig. 2.15 depicts the class "*Superficial fascia of male perineum*" (FMA20722), which is linked to the class "*Female body wall*" (FMA259159) through a sequence of 5 links. What makes this situation incorrect is the disjointness of the class at one end ("*Superficial fascia of male perineum*") with one at the other end ("*Female body wall*").

In order theory, the group of descendants of a class is called a "principal ideal." The systematic calculation of principal ideals involves transitive closure, which is computational prohibitive when multiple types of relations are involved. Therefore, to achieve a feasible PIE motifs implementation using SPARQL, we perform the computation in two phases. The first phase transforms the FMA OWL/XML source file by converting every *part-of* relational instance to an *is-a* instance. A relation-type-ignorant RDF store is created from this transformed source which encapsulates *structural, or hierarchical* information only

Table 2.7 The first 8 motifs accounts for all possible combinations of two relational types, *is-a* and *part-of*, between any pair among three classes. The remainder 4 motifs (9-12) represent configurations that fix any two relationships between *A*, *B* and *B*, *C*, but leaves the third one, between *A*, *C*, to be possibly disjoint. Disjointness exists between opposing gender classes, but may not be automatically inferred from antonyms

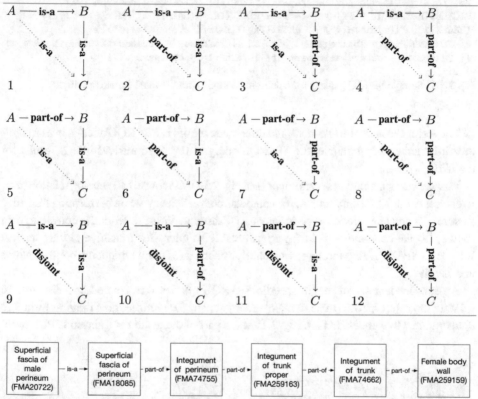

Fig. 2.15 The class "*Superficial fascia of male perineum*" (FMA20722) is linked to the class "*Female body wall*" (FMA259159) through a sequence of five *is-a* and *part-of* relationship instances

since directionality and linkage are maintained. The second phase involves look-ups, after interesting structural information is obtained, into a separate RDF store which faithfully encapsulates distinct relationships (which we use for two-node and three-node motifs). The second phase is used to query relational types necessary for detailed final results.

Implementation

The FMA OWL file was loaded into a Virtuoso RDF store, version 06.01.3127, hosted on a MacPro desktop machine with 32GB of RAM and one 2.8GHz Quad-Core Intel Xeon "Nehalem" processor, running Max OS X Snow Leopard [61]. The motif-specific SPARQL queries patterns were executed against the Virtuoso store using a simple script.

```
SELECT  distinct ?A ?B ?C  {
?A1 rdfs:label ?A .
?B1 rdfs:label ?B .
?C1 rdfs:label ?C .
?A1 rdfs:subClassOf ?B1.
?B1 rdfs:subClassOf [owl:onProperty ?a2bProp; owl:someValuesFrom ?C1].
FILTER((REGEX(?A, "[Ff]emale.*") && REGEX(?C, "(Male|[^e][Mm]ale).*")) ||
(REGEX(?C, "[Ff]emale.*") && REGEX(?A, "(Male|[^e][Mm]ale).*")))
FILTER(?a2bProp = obo:regional_part_of || ?a2bProp = obo:constitutional_part_of
|| ?a2bProp = obo:systemic_part_of || ?a2bProp = obo:part_of )  }
```

Fig. 2.16 Sample SPARQL query for a three-node motif with the male-female antonym

The script executed the two-node and three-node motifs in SPARQL queries in a straight-forward manner. For example, the SPARQL query in Fig. 2.16 retrieved the 9 results for motif 10.

PIE was implemented in several steps (see Fig. 2.17): (1) convert all *part-of* relation to *is-a* relation in the XML data source, for computational efficiency when performing transitive closure; (2) create a relation-type-ignorant RDF store in Virtuoso from the converted data source; (3) feed antonyms and (4) perform SPARQL query for transitive closure against Virtuoso's SPARQL API through a custom Ruby script; (5) output matching configurations in a csv file.

An independent set of length-specific SPARQL queries was created and executed to validate the result for the (male, female) antonym pair, for motif lengths ranging from 3 to 8, involving 4 to 9 nodes. In fact, Fig. 2.15 was a part of the result for a six-node PIE motif.

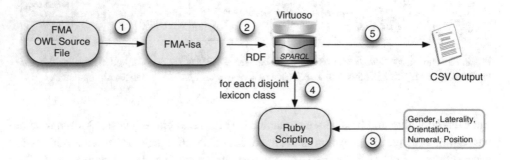

Fig. 2.17 PIE computational pipeline

2.4.2   Motifs Identified

For detailed results and analysis, please see [62]. This section briefly discusses the results obtained which are organized around the sizes of the motifs: two-node, three-node, and arbitrary-length motifs.

Two-Node Motifs
We found 180 pairs (A, B) such that A *is-a* B and also A is a *part-of* B (Type (I)); 330 cases where A *is-a* B, and A and B involve antonyms (Type (II)); and 130 cases where A is a *part-of* B, and A and B involve antonyms (Type (III)).

Three-Node Motifs
With a single edge relation linking three node classes, we considered 12 motifs as displayed in Table 2.7. Motifs 1-8 in Table 2.7 had 2,741 instances. The motifs 9-12 had 462 instances. Here, to capture "disjointness," we use antonyms as filters to track down a subset of class pairs that are more likely to be disjoint.

Arbitrary-Length Motifs
The PIE method exploits transitivity to identify subgraph patterns with an arbitrary number of links (Sect. 2.4.1). We have tested and validated PIE on FMA and found results beyond those captured by MOCH. It was discovered that in total there exists 755 root nodes with 4,100 respective descendants with opposing antonyms in their class names.

2.4.3   Findings

FMA
FMA is a large and complex ontological system, which currently consists of nearly 90,000 classes, over 174 spatio-structural relations, and about 2.4 million relationship instances. This section only addresses one aspect of quality assurance, though using an innovative approach whose results would be difficult to uncover through manual means de novo. We found it quite impressive that only a very small fraction of the FMA suffers from inconsistency and errors using our systematic motif checking. Such errors seem correctable without too much effort. Indeed, the Structural Informatics Group at UW is working on correcting the inconsistencies identified in this study.

Semantics of Part-of
Formal modeling of the semantics of the different kind of partonomy relationships is a well-recognized intricate topic [59]. It is especially challenging if logical reasoning is to be built on top of it [26]. From what we can learn from the denotational semantics of programming languages [63], there could be three general mechanisms to model the semantics of A is a *part-of* B at the class level: (a): $A \preceq_1 B$ if $(\forall x \in A)(\exists y \in B)\, p(x, y)$, where p is a binary relation at the instance level representing *part-of*; (b): $A \preceq_2 B$ if $(\forall y \in B)(\exists x \in A)\, p(y, x)$, where $p(y, x)$ reads "y *has-part* x;" (c): $A \preceq_3 B$ if both $A \preceq_1 B$ and $A \preceq_2 B$ hold. In terms

of the syntax of description logic, $A \preceq_1 B$ amounts to $A \sqsubseteq \exists pB$; $A \preceq_2 B$ amounts to $B \sqsubseteq \exists p^- A$; and $A \preceq_3 B$ amounts to $(A \sqsubseteq \exists pB) \sqcap (B \sqsubseteq \exists p^- A)$, where p^- is the reverse of p. The outcome of this study hinged upon interpretation (a), a standard semantic interpretation for *part-of*. To differentiate the meaning of the different partonomy relationships, one might consider such different possible interpretations. However, any change in interpretation is likely to impact the rest of the structure as well [59], and one needs to accept all logical consequences of any semantic commitment made.

Limitations

There are different versions of FMA and we did not systematically test our method on all of them for cross-validation. FMA is originally represented in a frame-based structure [64], which is not DL-based. Even though the OWL version of FMA we used is not semantically equivalent to its original representation, manual inspection with the version at http://fme. biostr.washington.edu:8080 shows that they share anomaly types identified here.

We have not studied motifs of a more complex structure beyond 3 nodes, other than the arbitrary-length linear motifs through PIE. However, such an investigation is entirely feasible based on our approach, as long as the complex-structured larger motifs capture patterns of interest.

Conclusion: Using Semantic Web-based techniques, we have successfully implemented MOCH and PIE for ontology quality assurance of FMA, specifically targeting the interaction of multiple types of relations captured as labeled graph motifs with disjointness constraints, in an exhaustive manner.

Our graph motif-based approach for ontology quality assurance has several unique aspects. First, arbitrarily sized motifs can be checked using PIE. Second, our approach has a rule-based, logical flavor, not only manifested in its implementation as "basic graph patterns" in SPARQL, but also in disjointness constraints between nodes. Third, our methodology and computational framework are completely general and are applicable to other ontological systems.

Additionally, the use of new advances in labeled motif analysis [65] can help characterize the label assignments on the edges of structurally equivalent small graph patterns to represent the distribution of the semantic information in those subgraphs in terms of joint link pattern to identify other anomalous patterns within the FMA. Finally, the IHSTDO (http://www.ihtsdo. org) has launched a project for reconstructing the anatomical ontology. Our method should remain applicable if OWL is used as the main representation mechanism, or a translation to OWL can be readily achieved.

2.5   Self-Bisimilarity

In this section, we introduce an auditing method that combines information from concepts and relations. We focus on symmetric concept pairs in the Foundational Model of Anatomy (FMA [58]), a commonly-used reference ontology in medicine. A pair of concepts is called

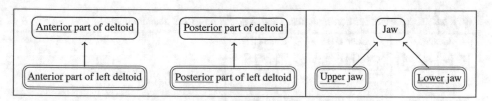

Fig. 2.18 The two ideal cases for bisimilar concepts. Arrows express the subsumption relationships in FMA

symmetric if the concept names are the same except for the possible difference in a single occurrence of symmetric modifiers used. For example, ("*Anterior part of deltoid*," "*Posterior part of deltoid* ") is a symmetric concept pair in FMA involving the modifier pair *anterior* and *posterior*. We propose the use of *bisimilarity* (a.k.a. bisimulation) for auditing symmetric concepts in FMA. Bisimulation is a technique used in Computer Science to capture similar behaviors in transition systems [66, 67]. We say that two concepts are *bisimilar* if: (1) they are symmetric; (2) their parents are either bisimilar or the same. We use the word "self-bisimilarity" to indicate the fact that the bisimilar concepts come from the same ontology.

The motivating idea for this work is that most symmetric concept pairs should be bisimilar, so the "symmetry" carries over to all ancestors of the respective pairs until a shared concept is reached. Figure 2.18 shows two example configurations, where the arrows express the subsumption relationships (*is-a*) in FMA.

In some cases, the expected symmetric counterparts of some concepts do not exist in the ontology, which may be an indication of missing concepts. For example, while "*Second toe*" exists in FMA, "*First toe*" does not. It was confirmed by FMA experts that "*First toe*" should also appear in FMA. Moreover, even when both symmetric concepts exist, they may not exhibit bisimilar structures as illustrated in Fig. 2.18. This can be seen from Fig. 2.19: the symmetric pair (*Upper lip proper*, *Lower lip proper*) exists in FMA, however, they do not share a parent concept: "Lower lip proper " is not classified as a subclass of "*Subdivision of mouth*" in FMA, which represents a misaligned relationship.

This section provides a comprehensive study of substructures associated with symmetric concepts. We divide symmetric concept pairs into two groups:

Fig. 2.19 An example of abnormal structure. Dashed arrow indicates the absence of subsumption relationship between the nodes

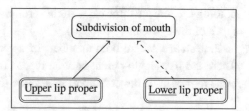

Table 2.8 Three cases for non-matches. Shaded nodes represent absent concepts

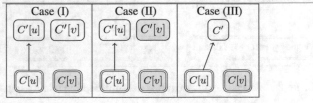

Table 2.9 Five types for matches. Shaded nodes represent absent concepts. Dashed arrows represent missing *is-a* relationships

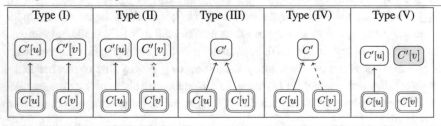

Table 2.10 The eight patterns of mixed parent contexts for problematic Matches. Shaded nodes represent absent concepts. Dashed arrows represent missing *is-a* relationships

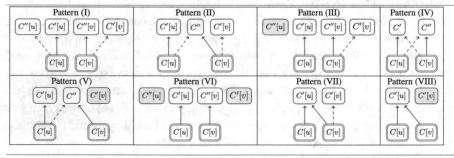

1. *Non-Matches*, where only one member of a symmetric concept pair appears in the ontology. There are three cases in this group, distinguished by the possible appearances and types of their parents (Table 2.8).

2. *Matches*, where both members of a symmetric concept pair appear in the ontology. There are five single-parent-context types (Table 2.9) and eight mixed-parent-context patterns representing the combination of these five types (Table 2.10).

2.5.1   Auditing Approach for Symmetric Concepts

A concept name can be divided into two parts: A modifier and a context which is the remaining string apart from the modifier. We use u, v to represent modifiers and use C to represent context. $C[u]$ then represents the concept name comprised of C and u, similarly with $C[v]$. Taking different modifiers and different positions of the modifiers into account, one concept name may have multiple divisions. For example, *"Lumen of anterior ramus of right anterior segmental bronchus"* has two divisions for the modifier *"anterior"*: *"Lumen of anterior ramus of right anterior segmental bronchus"* and *"Lumen of anterior ramus of right anterior segmental bronchus,"* where the underlined modifier is the one focused on.

We use pair (u, v) to represent symmetric modifiers. Putting the symmetric modifiers into the same context C results in a symmetric concept pair $(C[u], C[v])$. As a result, the above concept *"Lumen of anterior ramus of right anterior segmental bronchus"* has two symmetric concepts: *"Lumen of posterior ramus of right anterior segmental bronchus"* and *"Lumen of anterior ramus of right posterior segmental bronchus."*

More than 80% of the concepts in FMA contain modifiers in their names. We provide an automatic approach to extract all the symmetric modifier pairs in FMA and rank them by their occurrences (The specific steps will be explained in Section 3.3). Six pairs of them are selected for further analysis.

Non-matches

For a symmetric concept pair, if only the first member appears in the ontology, it is called a Non-Match. For example, for the pair *(Pleura of lower lobe of left lung, Pleura of upper lobe of left lung)*, the first member appears in FMA and the second one does not. In this scenario, it is natural to trace back to the ancestors to investigate the original reason. As illustrated in the left diagram of Fig. 2.20, we discover a concept *"Pleura of lower lobe of left lung"* whose symmetric concept *"Pleura of upper lobe of left lung"* is absent in FMA.

When investigating its parent *"Pleura of lower lobe,"* we discover that the parent's symmetric concept *"Pleura of upper lobe"* does exist. So the question is: why does *"Pleura of upper lobe of left lung"* not exist, and why is it not a child of *"Pleura of upper lobe?"* This kind of scenario is captured by Case (I) in Table 2.8.

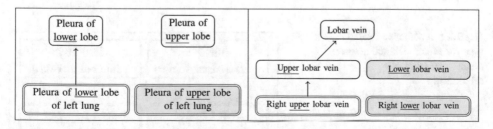

Fig. 2.20 (1) Example of Case (I) in Table 2.8; (2) A Non-Match trace. Shaded nodes represent absent concepts

Note that in our diagrams, we always use the solid arrow "$\longrightarrow$" to represent the *is-a* relationship *rdfs:subClassOf*. A dashed arrow "$--\rightarrow$" means that the *is-a* relationship is missing between the head and tail, and a shaded node indicates that the corresponding concept does not appear in FMA at all.

There are two other cases for Non-Matches, as illustrated by Case (II) and Case (III) in Table 2.8, the details on all the cases are explained in the following:

- Case (I): $C[u]$ exists in FMA while $C[v]$ does not. The parent of $C[u]$ also contains the modifier u but with a different context C', and $C'[v]$ is a concept existing in FMA.
- Case (II): $C[u]$ exists in FMA while $C[v]$ does not. The parent of $C[u]$ also contains the modifier u but with a different context C'. The same as $C[v]$, $C'[v]$ does not exist in FMA.
- Case (III): $C[u]$ exists in FMA while $C[v]$ does not, and the parent of $C[u]$ does not contain the modifier u.

By looking into those cases we can discover that (II) is the only consistent case: the fact that $C[v]$ does not exist in FMA is caused by the nonexistence of $C'[v]$ in FMA. If tracing back along Case (II) to their ancestors, we can always reach Case (I) or Case (III). For example, in the right diagram of Fig. 2.20, by tracing back two steps, we reach Case (III). As a result, there exist clustered Non-Match trees where the roots belong to Case (I) or Case (III) while all the other nodes belong to Case (II). These kinds of roots are called *Non-Match tree roots*. While every pair in Case (II) must be a node in some tree, many pairs in Case (I) or Case (III) are just isolated nodes since they do not have any Non-Match descendant. As we can see, the tree roots help domain experts to limit and focus their effort when auditing ontologies.

If $C[u]$ appears as a concept name in FMA, $C[v]$ is supposed to be a concept name in FMA as well, and vice versa. When both $C[u]$ and $C[v]$ are concept names in FMA for some context C, the pair $(C[u], C[v])$ is called a Match. If we trace back to their parents, then ideally, there are supposed to be two cases, as illustrated by the examples in Fig. 2.18 in Section 1: (1) Their parents are also a Match and contain the same modifiers with their children separately; (2) They share the same parent which does not contain the modifier u or v at all.

Fig. 2.21 Another abnormal type for Match. Dashed arrow means a missing *is-a* relationship

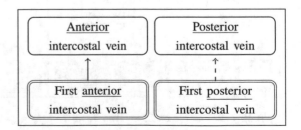

Matches

Even though most of the Matches in FMA maintain good bisimilar structures, there still exist abnormalities. The example shown in Fig. 2.19 in Section 1 is only one such case. There are more abnormal structures on Matches. For example, there is a Match (*First anterior inter-costal vein, First posterior intercostal vein*), where *"First anterior intercostal vein"* has parent *"Anterior intercostal vein."* Although the symmetric concept for *"Anterior inter-costal vein"* exists in FMA, it does not have *"First posterior intercostal vein"* as its child, as shown in Fig. 2.21. This scenario is captured by Type (II) in Table 2.9.

For Matches, when considering only single parent context, we can classify all of them into five types, as shown in Table 2.9.

- Type (I): The parent of $C[u]$ also contains the modifier u but with a different context C', $C'[v]$ also exists in FMA with $C[v]$ being a sub-class of $C'[v]$.
- Type (II): The parent of $C[u]$ also contains the modifier u but with a different context C', $C'[v]$ also exists in FMA, but $C[v]$ is not a sub-class of $C'[v]$.
- Type (III): The parent of $C[u]$ does not contain the modifier u, and $C[u]$ and $C[v]$ share the same parent.
- Type (IV): The parent of $C[u]$ does not contain the modifier u, but $C[u]$ and $C[v]$ do not share the same parent.
- Type (V): The parent of $C[u]$ also contains the modifier u but with a different context C', but $C'[v]$ does not exist at all.

It is clear that Type (I) is an ideal case. For Type (III), it is an ideal case when the parent C' does not contain the modifier v neither. Other types indicate potential errors in the modeling procedure.

Patterns for Abnormal Matches   The calculation of the above five types is unilateral, i.e, it only considers single-parent context. For those problematic non-symmetric ones (Type (II), (IV), and (V)), the type of $(C[v], C[u])$ may be different from that of $(C[u], C[v])$. As a result, there are nine mixed combinations, resulting in six different patterns considering the fact that some of them have symmetric structures. They are illustrated in Table 2.10 from Pattern (I) to Pattern (VI).

Besides the six patterns, there are two more patterns that can be easily ignored. As stated before, in Type (III) (Table 2.9), the parent C' does not contain the modifier u, but may contain the modifier v. In that case, if we change the order of the members in the pair, the resulting type can be Type (II) or Type(V). For example, as illustrated in the left diagram of Fig. 2.22, *"C8 part of]posterior division of brachial plexus"* is a child of *"Branch of anterior ramus of eighth cervical nerve"* instead of *"Branch of posterior ramus of eighth cervical nerve"* even though the latter one exists in FMA. In this case, from right to left, it is Type (III), but from left to right, the type is changed to Type (II). In another example, as shown in the right diagram of Fig. 2.22, the type is Type (III) from right to left and is changed to Type (V) after we change the order of the members in the pair. As a result, we need to

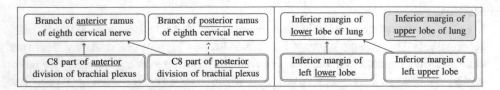

Fig. 2.22 (1) Example of Pattern (VII); (2) Example of Pattern (VIII). Shaded nodes represent absent concepts. Dashed arrows represent missing *is-a* relationships

add Pattern (VII) and Pattern (VIII) to Table 2.10. Although pairs in these two patterns are rare, we still need to list them in order to be theoretically complete.

The eight patterns we presented above provide the human editors of biomedical ontologies a full dimensional view of all the structures for Matches, which can be helpful in discovering and introducing new ontology design patterns [68, 69].

Implementation

The FMA OWL file was loaded into a Virtuoso RDF store [61], version 06.01.3127, hosted on a MacPro desktop machine with 32GB of RAM and one 2.8GHz Quad-Core Intel Xeon "Nehalem" processor, running Mac OS X Snow Leopard.

In order to retrieve all the modifier pairs, we first obtained all the class names in FMA and used Natural Language Processing (NLP) methods to obtain all the Noun-Phrase (NP) chunks without prepositions. As a result, 22510 NP chunks were obtained. Then we retrieved all the modifier pairs in which the two members shared common contexts from the chunks. Finally, we ranked the pairs by the number of common contexts their members share. The first twenty pairs we obtained are: *(left, right), (anterior, posterior), (superior, inferior), (lateral,medial), (first, second), (second, third), (first, third), (fourth, third), (fourth, second), (lateral, anterior), (first, fourth), (lower, upper), (fourth, fifth), (third, fifth), (deep, superficial), (second, fifth), (first,fifth), (posterior, lateral), (external, internal), (fourth,sixth).*

We selected five pairs from the first twenty pairs and another pair from the rest for experiment. For each input symmetric modifier pair (u, v), we employed an algorithm of the following steps:

1. Query the RDF database, obtain all the concept names containing the modifier u, and their divisions on u;
2. Replace u in each division with v, query the database again to see if the symmetric concept exists; obtain all the Matches and Non-Matches from u to v;
3. Change u and v into each other, repeat step 1 and step 2; obtain all the Non-Matches from v to u;
4. For all the Matches between u and v, query the information of their parents, then divide them into the five types in Table 2.9;
5. Check mixed parent context information for those problematic pairs from the above step, then divide them into the eight patterns in Table 2.10;

6. For Non-Matches from u to v, query the information of their parents; divide them into the three cases in Table 2.8, and obtain all the Non-Match tree roots;

7. For Non-Matches from v to u, query the information of their parents; divide them into the three cases in Table 2.8, and obtain all the Non-Match tree roots.

One thing needs to be noted in our algorithm: When checking whether the concept contains the same modifier as its parent do to decide the types in Table 2.9, if the modifier occurs multiple times in the term, context information around it has to be used. In our experiment, we use the words before and after the modifier as the helpers: if both modifiers in the parent and the child share the same words before or after them, they are treated as the same modifier. For example, *"Parenchyma of anterior part of right anterior bronchopulmonary subsegment"* has parent *"Parenchyma of anterior part of anterior bronchopulmonary subsegment."* When the first *anterior* is in question, to confirm that the parent contains the same modifier, context information *"Parenchyma of "* was used. When the second *anterior* is in question, the other context information *"bronchopulmonary subsegment"* was used.

2.5.2 Errors Detected by the Method

In this section, we briefly discuss the results obtained by this method. For detailed results and analysis, please see [70].

After applying our automatic method for extracting modifiers in FMA, we discovered 1304 pairs of modifiers in which both members have at least 10 common contexts, and 34 pairs of modifiers in which both members have at least 100 common contexts. Six pairs of them that are most commonly used and most intuitively to introduce bisimilar concepts were selected for further experimentation: *(left, right), (anterior, posterior), (first, second), (superior, inferior), (upper, lower), (ascending, descending)*.

Non-matches
It was seen that, more than half of the concepts whose names contain the modifier *"posterior"* do not have their symmetric concepts appearing in FMA. On the other hand, it is remarkable that for the pair *(left, right)*, there are only about 5% of Non-Matches. For others, the percentages of Non-Matches are between 10% to 35%.

It was seen that, there existed 9893 Non-Matches with 1219 Non-Match tree roots totally. Except for the pair *(left, right)*, Case (II) occupies more than 50%, which is reasonable due to the fact that Case (II) is the consequence of Case (I) or Case (III). Although Case (II) occupies a large part of the Non-Matches, after clustering, the number of trees they belong to is reduced dramatically. This limits the effort of domain experts since they can focus on auditing the tree roots.

Except for tree roots, other pairs in Case (I) and Case (III) are isolated Non-Matches. For example, more than 75% of Non-Matches for the pair *(left, right)* are in Case (III). While there are only a few tree roots for this case, we can conclude that most of the pairs are isolated Non-Matches.

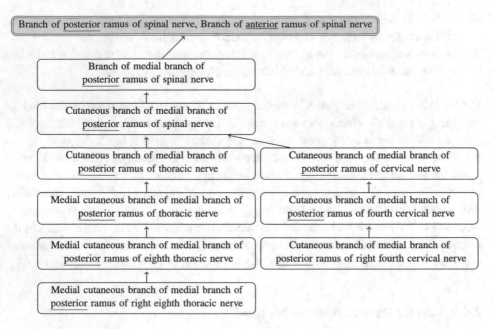

Fig. 2.23 The node in pink contains a symmetric concept pair. All descendants of it are Non-Matches with their corresponding symmetric concepts missing, where "Branch of medial branch of posterior ramus of spinal nerve" is the tree root

Figure 2.23 illustrates part of a tree with the tree root *"Branch of medial branch of posterior ramus of spinal nerve"* in Case (I). All descendants of the root have their corresponding symmetric concepts missing in FMA. It is clear that the absence of *"Branch of medial branch of anterior ramus of spinal nerve"* causes the absence of the other eight symmetric concepts for other descendants.

Matches

It was seen that there exist 221 abnormal Matches. These occupied a negligible portion of all the Matches (less than 4%), which in turn confirmed our intuition that Type (I) and (III) are ideal situations. Among the eight patterns for abnormal Matches, Pattern (IV) turns out to be the most common one with 151 instances, where the parents for the two symmetric concepts are two different contexts.

2.5.3   Manual Evaluation of the Results

Manual evaluation was conducted by FMA experts from the Structural Informatics Group of the University of Washington, where the latest version of FMA is managed and maintained.

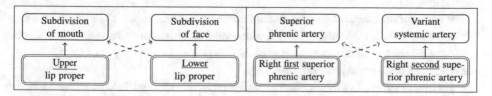

Fig. 2.24 Two detected error examples among the abnormal matches

Non-matches

Among the 9893 Non-Matches discovered by our algorithm, we randomly selected 176 tree roots for evaluation. Manual inspection confirmed that 58% of them are missing concepts that need to be or already has been added to the latest version of FMA.

Matches

All the 221 abnormal Matches in were evaluated by FMA experts. 40 true errors were found among them, including one deprecated term and 4 terms with misspellings. Figure 2.24 illustrates two examples that were identified by FMA experts as true errors: for the example on the left, both *"Upper lip proper"* and *"Lower lip proper"* should have the same parent *"Lip proper;"* for the example on the right, both children should have the same parent *"Superior phrenic artery."*

Recall the two examples in Fig. 2.22, it was pointed out by domain experts that the parent assignments for the example on the left is correct. However, for the example on the right of Fig. 2.22, *"Inferior margin of left upper lobe"* should have parent *"Inferior margin of upper lobe of lung,"* which was already implemented in the current version of FMA.

2.5.4   Analysis of False Positives and Other Limitations of the Method

The fact that there are false positive results among the Non-Matches and misaligned Matches discovered by our method is due to the traditional convention used in naming FMA concepts in tree structures such as arteries, veins, nerves, and lymphatic trees. For example, *"Left diagonal artery"* is actually the diagonal branch of *"left coronary artery."* There is no diagonal branch for the *"right coronary artery,"* hence no *"right diagonal artery."* Another example for Matches: the class *"Superior epigastric artery"* is a branch (subtree) of *"Internal thoracic artery,"* hence has the parent class *"Subdivision of internal thoracic artery;"* while on the other hand, the class *"Inferior epigastric artery"* is a branch of *"External iliac artery proper,"* hence the child of *"Subdivision of external iliac artery proper."* If we were to classify them based solely on location (epigastrium), then we would create a class called *"Epigastric artery"* which would then subsume both the superior and inferior types. However the location attribute as the primary axis for classification does not add more meaningful information or knowledge about the arteries.

For each symmetric concept pair, when defining the cases, types and patterns, we only look up to the parents without going down to the children at the same time, which might seem insufficient. However, if we switch to the children's point of view, they become parents. So, it is not necessary to consider both directions.

Only binary symmetric modifiers are considered in this section. To deal with non-binary relations such as (anterior, medial, lateral), one solution is to treat them pairwise, while the other solution is to treat them holistically. For the latter solution, we first need to extend Matches and Non-Matches from pairs to arrays, then define all the types and cases for them accordingly. However, it is predictable that the numbers of those types and cases will increase exponentially since all the possible combinations have to be taken into account. As a result, treating the non-binary relations pairwise and then combining the results may be a more feasible route.

Conclusion: We proposed a principled ontology auditing approach based on structural bisimilarity, and provided exhaustive analysis on six prominent modifier pairs. A significant amount of previously unknown errors were discovered and have been incorporated into the latest version of FMA. The uniqueness of our structural auditing method lies in three aspects. First, instead of manually providing the symmetric modifier pairs, we automatically compute all the pairs from FMA and rank them. Second, our methodology stems from the bisimulation theory in Computer Science. Different from randomly choosing some isolated structures for analysis, as is typical in the literature, the cases, types, and patterns we define are theoretically complete. Third, we not only discover those concepts with high likelihood of errors, but also point out the roots where the errors were introduced. The eight patterns for the problematic Matches also help the domain experts trace back to the original conceptual errors, which can be useful in discovering and creating new design patterns in the processes of creating new ontologies [71, 68, 69].

We applied our methodology to the legacy version of FMA from the OBO foundry [72]. The algorithm we proposed is scalable and can be easily applied to other versions of FMA or other ontologies. Except for *is-a*, the *part-of* relationship can be brought into the picture in our future work. The most prominent difference between *is-a* and *part-of* relationships is that in the former, each concept can only have one parent in FMA, and in the latter, each concept can have multiple parents. Thus, the analysis of the *part-of* relationship will require more complex structures.

For detailed results and analysis, please see [70].

Formal Concept Analysis and Semantic Completeness

3

Biomedical terminologies have been increasingly used in modern biomedical research and applications to facilitate data management and ensure semantic interoperability. As part of the evolution process, new concepts are regularly added to biomedical terminologies in response to the evolving domain knowledge and emerging applications. Most existing concept enrichment methods suggest new concepts via directly importing knowledge from external sources. In this chapter, we investigate formal concept analysis (FCA) to identify potentially missing concepts in a given terminology by leveraging its intrinsic knowledge – concept names and their definitions.

3.1 Missing Concepts

In this section, we introduce a lexical- and FCA-based method to identify potentially missing concepts in the NCI Thesaurus. Lexical features (i.e., words appeared in the concept names) are considered as FCA attributes while generating formal context. Applying multistage intersection of FCA attributes identifies newly formalized bags of words (i.e., FCA formal concepts) that represent missing concepts, which may be further validated through external knowledge.

3.1.1 The Lexical- and FCA-Based Approach

Our method mainly consists of two steps: (1) pre-processing concept names and constructing FCA formal context; and (2) performing FCA via a multistage intersection algorithm to identify potentially missing (or new) concepts in the NCI Thesaurus.

© The Author(s), under exclusive license to Springer Nature Switzerland AG 2022
G.-Q. Zhang et al., *Formal Methods for the Analysis of Biomedical Ontologies*,
Synthesis Lectures on Data, Semantics, and Knowledge,
https://doi.org/10.1007/978-3-031-12131-9_3

Constructing Formal Context

Given a collection of concepts in the terminology, we consider all the concepts as FCA objects O and words appearing in the concept names (i.e., lexical features) as FCA attributes A, respectively. With the binary relation $R \subseteq O \times A$ specifying whether concept $o \in O$ contains word $a \in A$, we can construct the FCA formal context $K = (O, A, R)$.

Since words appearing in concept names may have variations (e.g., plural versus singular forms) or synonyms, we perform attribute/word normalization to create a more robust FCA formal context. For word variations, we normalize words appearing in concept names using LuiNorm [73], a lexical tool provided by the UMLS. For example, "bones" can be normalized to "bone." Regarding word synonyms, we leverage concepts in the NCI Thesaurus with single-word preferred names and single-word synonyms. More specifically, if a word w itself is the preferred name of an NCI Thesaurus concept and has a synonym s that is also a single word, then we maintain a mapping between the synonym s and the preferred name w. This way, words with the same meanings can be normalized to their preferred names thus the same attribute.

Identifying Potentially Missing Concepts

To derive FCA formal concepts, we leverage the idea of the faster concept analysis introduced in [74], which is to perform multistage intersection on each pair of formal concepts from the initial formal concept set consisting of all objects, until no more new formal concept is generated. The pseudocode of the algorithm is shown in Algorithm 1.

Algorithm 1: Pseudocode of identifying potentially missing concepts by multistage intersection.

---

1 **Input:** Formal context (O, A, R)
2 **Output:** Missing concept set M
3 **Initialization:**
4 Original set $S_O \leftarrow \{o^\uparrow | o \in O\}$
5 Initial set $I \leftarrow S_O$
6 Newly derived formal concept set $N \leftarrow S_O$
7 **while** $N \neq 0$ **do**
8   Last iteration formal concept set $L \leftarrow I$
9   **for** *each pair* (C_x, C_y) *in* L **do**
10   I.add(Intersection(C_x, C_y))
11   **end**
12      $N \leftarrow (I - L)$
13 **end**
14 $M \leftarrow I - S_O$

In practice, for computation convenience, we perform operations on the lexical feature sets (i.e., using FCA attribute sets to represent FCA formal concepts). The initial set of FCA formal concepts is a set of FCA attribute sets, that is, the lexical feature sets of all the original concepts (i.e., $\{o^\uparrow \mid o \in O\}$). In the first iteration, we compute the intersection of each pair of FCA attribute sets in the initial set; and if the result is not included in the initial set, we add it into the initial set. We repeat this process until no new FCA attribute set can be derived.

Each newly generated FCA attribute set is taken as the lexical feature set of a potentially missing concept among the given concepts. An advantage of using lexical features (or words) as FCA attribute sets is that these words can be further leverage to name the newly discovered concepts.

Illustrative Example

Figure 3.1 shows a simple example of FCA formal context in a tabular format generated from the concept *Breast Fibroepithelial Neoplasm* (C40405) and its descendants in the NCI Thesaurus. The cells with check marks represent the binary relation between the concepts and their lexical features. Note that the word "Tumor" is normalized to "neoplasm," since it is a synonym of *Neoplasm* (C3262) in the NCI Thesaurus.

Given the FCA formal context, the FCA formal concept with attribute set {breast, neoplasm} (see blue cells in Fig. 3.1) can be derived by intersecting the attribute sets of "*Borderline Breast Phyllodes Tumor*" (C5316) and "*Breast Fibroepithelial Neoplasm*" (C40405). Therefore, a concept with lexical feature set {breast, neoplasm} is considered as a potentially missing concept for the given FCA formal context. This example only intends to illustrate

	juvenile	fibroepithelial	malignant	breast	fibroadenoma	neoplasm	complex	borderline	pericanalicular	intracanalicular	benign	phyllode	giant
C3744: Breast Fibroadenoma				✓	✓								
C7575: Breast Phyllodes Tumor				✓		✓						✓	
C4271: Breast Intracanalicular Fibroadenoma				✓	✓					✓			
C4272: Breast pericanalicular Fibroadenoma				✓	✓				✓				
C4273: Breast Giant Fibroadenoma				✓	✓								✓
C4276: Breast Juvenile Fibroadenoma	✓			✓	✓								
C5194: Breast Complex Fibroadenoma				✓	✓		✓						
C4504: Malignant Breast Phyllodes Tumor			✓	✓		✓						✓	
C5196: Benign Breast Phyllodes Tumor				✓		✓					✓	✓	
C5316: Borderline Breast Phyllodes Tumor				✓		✓		✓				✓	
C40405: Breast Fibroepithelial Neoplasm		✓		✓		✓							

Fig. 3.1 An example of FCA formal context generated by the concept "*Breast Fibroepithelial Neoplasm*" (C40405) in the NCI Thesaurus and its descendants in company with their lexical features. Word "Tumor" is normalized to "neoplasm" and word "Phyllodes" is normalized to "phyllode." An FCA formal concept (marked by blue cells) with FCA attribute set {breast, neoplasm} is considered as a potentially missing concept among the given concepts

how our method works, and one may have noticed that *"Breast Neoplasm"* (C2910) is an existing concept in the NCI Thesaurus although it is not among the given concepts. For the actual implementation of our method, we further check if the newly generated concepts are existing in the NCI Thesaurus and ensure the removal of such cases from the list of potentially missing concepts.

3.1.2   Overall Results and the Preliminary Evaluation

We applied our method to the sub-hierarchies under *"Disease or Disorder"* (C2991) in the NCI Thesaurus (19.08d version) and identified 8,983 potential missing concepts.

We performed a preliminary evaluation to validate the potentially missing concepts identified using the external knowledge in the UMLS. For each potentially missing concept identified, we checked whether its lexical feature set could be matched to any concept name from the external terminologies in the UMLS. We found 592 out of 8,983 potentially missing concepts are included in the external terminologies in UMLS. For detailed results and analysis, please see [75].

3.1.3   Limitations of This Approach

This work has several limitations that need further improvement. First, the potentially missing concepts detected by our method may not be directly imported into a terminology. This is because different terminologies are developed for disparate purposes and have varying target applications, and a concept that is essential for a terminology may not be necessary for another. Further reviews and evaluations by the terminology curators are still required to decide whether a concept is meaningful and should be added according to the scope of the terminology and its potential applications.

A limitation of using words in concept names as the FCA attributes is that the "subconcept-superconcept" relation derived may be different from the hierarchical *is-a* relation in the original terminology. For instance, *"Breast Neoplasm"* and *"Breast"* are two new concepts generated based on the FCA formal context in Fig. 3.1. Although the two concepts have a "subconcept-superconcept" relation in terms of the FCA word attributes, they do not form a valid *is-a* relation. In fact, *"Breast"* is located in a different sub-hierarchy *Organ*. A potential solution to avoid such cases is to use enriched lexical features for a concept, which includes its ancestor's lexical features. This way, the original hierarchical relation will be captured in the initial FCA formal context, and thus the new concepts generated by attribute set intersection will locate within the same sub-hierarchy with the root concept. However, the enriched lexical features may make it more difficult to decide which words to use for naming a concept. To deal with this, we plan to leverage both logical definitions and lexical features to identify and name missing concepts.

Conclusion: In this section, we introduced a lexical- and FCA-based method that utilizes intrinsic knowledge of a terminology to detect potentially missing concepts. We applied our method to the NCI Thesaurus *Disease or Disorder* sub-hierarchy and identified 8,983 potentially missing concepts. The preliminary evaluation via external validation using UMLS showed encouraging evidence for the effectiveness of our method.

3.2 Semantic Completeness

The completeness of a medical terminology system consists of two parts: complete content coverage and complete semantics. In this section, we focus on semantic completeness and present a scalable approach, called Spark-MCA, for evaluating the semantic completeness of SNOMED CT. To study semantic completeness, Jiang and Chute [76] used Formal Concept Analysis (FCA) as a tool to construct contexts from normal form presentations in SNOMED CT and analyzed the resulting lattice hierarchy for unlabeled nodes. These unlabeled nodes signify semantically incomplete areas in SNOMED CT which can serve as the candidate pool of new concepts for inclusion in SNOMED CT.

Most existing algorithms for computing formal concepts are not scalable to very large contexts. The process of generating formal concept hierarchies and constructing concept lattices from large contexts, after formal concepts are identified, is an additional computationally costly step. Due to such challenges, no scalable approaches have been proposed to exhaustively audit the semantic completeness of large biomedical ontologies using FCA, even with the aid of cloud computing technology. To address the computational challenge involved in constructing concept lattices from large contexts, we propose Spark-MCA, a Spark-based Multistage algorithm for Concept Analysis. Spark-MCA implements our proposed new FCA-based algorithms within the Apache Spark distributed cloud computing framework to provide a scalable approach for exhaustively analyzing the semantic completeness of large biomedical ontologies.

There are two basic algorithmic strategies for computing formal concepts: (a) forming intersections by joining one attribute at a time, and (b) repeatedly forming pairwise intersections starting from the attribute concepts. Kuznetsov and Obiedkov provided a survey and comparative evaluation of algorithms for FCA [77]. Bordat [78] used strategy (a), while Chein [79] used strategy (b). In this study, we use the idea of Troy, Zhang, Tian's [74] multistage algorithm for constructing concept lattices (MCA) and adapt and extend it in order to take advantage of the scalable distributed Spark framework.

We use ontological definitions for constructing a formal context. One can think of ontological concepts as objects, and ontological relationships as attributes in constructing a formal context. For example, with respect to Fig. 3.2 we can use [69483009 |*Shunt of cerebral ventricle to extracranial site (procedure)*|] as an object and the other lines as its attribute entries.

3.2.1   Spark-Based Multistage Algorithm for Concept Analysis

Overview

In this section, we introduce Spark-MCA, a distributed algorithm based on MCA, using the theoretical basis of FCA and adapting it to the Spark framework. Spark-MCA contains two parts: distributed MCA for obtaining all concepts, and distributed big set operation for lattice diagram construction. Spark-MCA takes in the original concepts and relations from SNOMED CT as source formal context and generates the entire concept lattice. We illustrate the main steps of our algorithm in the following subsections with the help of an example dataset extracted from SNOMED CT (Fig. 3.3).

We performed two types of evaluation: (1) partial validity, and (2) computational performance. To demonstrate that our Spark-MCA can be used in auditing semantic completeness and the results of our algorithm can provide a viable candidate pool of new concepts in a developing ontological system, we apply Retrospective Ground-Truthing (RGT) (discussed in Sect. 7.2) by comparing the results of Spark-MCA with the concepts added to SNOMED CT versions. For computational performance, we tested our algorithm for its scalability by comparing the running times for datasets of different sizes. We also evaluated our algorithm on its performance on the same dataset but using different numbers of working computer processors.

Model SNOMED CT Using the FCA

SNOMED CT uses name-value to describe composite expressions. Take the following in Fig. 3.2 as an example.

405813007 | *Procedure site—Direct (attribute)* |→ 35764002 | *Brain ventricle structure (body structure)* Here, 405813007 | *Procedure site—Direct (attribute)* | is the name part, while 35764002 | *Brain ventricle structure (body structure)* is the value part. We use

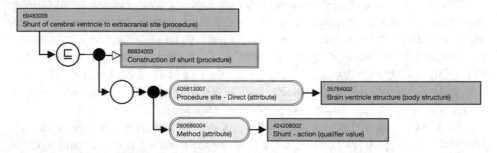

Fig. 3.2 SNOMED CT concept expression for *"Shunt of cerebral ventricle to extracranial site."*

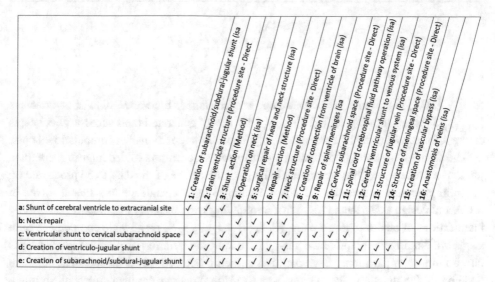

	1: Creation of subarachnoid/subdural-jugular shunt (isa	2: Brain ventricle structure (Procedure site - Direct)	3: Shunt action (Method)	4: Operation on neck (isa)	5: Surgical repair of head and neck structure (isa)	6: Repair - action (Method)	7: Neck structure (isa)	8: Creation of connection from ventricle of brain (isa)	9: Repair of spinal meninges (isa	10: Cervical subarachnoid space (Procedure site - Direct)	11: Spinal cord cerebrospinal fluid pathway operation (isa)	12: Cerebral ventricular shunt to venous system (isa)	13: Structure of jugular vein (Procedure site - Direct)	14: Structure of meningeal space (Procedure site - Direct)	15: Creation of vascular bypass (isa)	16: Anastomosis of veins (isa)
a: Shunt of cerebral ventricle to extracranial site	✓	✓	✓													
b: Neck repair				✓	✓	✓	✓									
c: Ventricular shunt to cervical subarachnoid space	✓	✓	✓	✓	✓	✓	✓	✓	✓	✓	✓					
d: Creation of ventriculo-jugular shunt	✓	✓	✓	✓	✓	✓	✓						✓	✓	✓	
e: Creation of subarachnoid/subdural-jugular shunt	✓	✓	✓	✓	✓	✓	✓							✓	✓	✓

Fig. 3.3 An example formal context in SNOMED CT

two steps to construct a formal concept from such SNOMED CT expressions. First, we include SNOMED CT concepts objects and each of their name-value pair as one attribute. For example, Fig. 3.2 is encoded as 69483009: 116680003 → 88834003; 405813007 → 35764002; 260686004 → 424208002, where we used identifiers for simplicity. Second, to enrich the attributes, we include its ancestors' attributes by leverage transitive closure of the *is-a* relation (identifier 116680003). With the second step, Fig. 3.2 is encoded as 69483009: 116680003 → 138875005; 405813007 → 35764002; 260686004 → 424208002; 26068 6004 → 129264002, where 138875005 is the root of the sub-hierarchy and dose not have any ancestors.

Spark-MCA
Algorithm for Distributed MCA
The distributed part of Spark-MCA is built on top of MCA [74]. The idea behind MCA is to perform multistage intersection operations on each pair of concepts from the initial concept set consisting of all objects, until no more new concept is generated. Each of the stages is independent of the previous ones and does not involve any concepts in the previous stages. For notational preparation, define $S \pitchfork T := \{s \cap t | s \in S, t \in T\}$, where S and T are collections of subsets. With respect to a given formal context (X, Y, R), the MCA algorithm involves the following iterative steps:

$$S_0 := \{X\},$$
$$S_1 := \{\{x\}^\uparrow | x \in X\}, \text{ and}$$
$$S_{i+1} := (S_i \cap S_i) - \bigcup_{1 \le k \le i} S_k$$

for $i \ge 1$. One important intermediate step for each stage is to remove all existing concepts $\bigcup_{1 \le k \le i} S_k$ when forming S_{i+1}. This way, only newly generated (and necessary) concepts are kept for subsequent stages, resulting in potentially large savings in computational cost.

The strategy involved in designing a distributed algorithm is to decompose a complex job into a sequence of jobs and to distribute particular parts of the data to be processed on different processing nodes. Our idea is to leverage the independence of stages involved in MCA and design a distributed MCA in the following way: Instead of iteratively performing intersections of object concepts pairs, $(S_i \cap S_i) - \bigcup_{1 \le k \le i} S_k$ on a single computer in each stage, we employ the MapReduce paradigm to split the iteration of pairwise intersections into a number of partitions. Each partition is then processed on an independent compute node by a *Map* function. The outputs from the *Map* functions are then collected, shuffled, and sent to compute nodes to perform *Reduce* functions. The output of *Reduce* functions are split again to repeat the steps above. While iterations involved in MapReduce become very expensive in a standard Hadoop MapReduce implementation due to the I/O latency between the MapReduce steps, the distributed MCA implemented using the Spark framework can take advantage of in-memory processing to reduce the I/O latency.

Algorithm 2: Distributed MCA

   Data: Formal context (X, Y, R)
   Result: Formal concept set C
1 initialize $S = \{x^\uparrow | x \in X)$
2 *candidate* $= S$
3 **while** $|candidate| > 1$ **do**
4 $\quad$ *canditade* $= \emptyset$
5 $\quad$ $Pair < Int, Int > = S.combination(S)$
6 $\quad$ **Function** $Map(p \in Pair)$
7 $\quad\quad$ $RDD< Int, Int > c = (p_{.1} \wedge p_{.2}, 1)$
8 $\quad$ **Function** $Reduce((c, 1))$
9 $\quad\quad$ *candidate* $= collect(c)$
10 $\quad$ $C = \bigcup candidate$
11 **end**
12 **return** C

Data in Spark are generally represented in the form of MapReduce key-value pairs $<k, v>$ and stored as resilient distributed datasets (RDDs). Algorithm 2 describes the concept formation phase in Spark-MCA to generate all concepts from a given context. First we initialize the primitive concept set using $S = \{x^\uparrow | x \in X\}$. Then, each loop in the *while* block (lines 3–11) performs one pairwise intersection. In each iterative step, we first obtain all pairs of current concepts as the *keys* for the input to *Map* (line 5). Then we split the pairs into a number of partitions and send them to compute node. Every node performs *Map* tasks of intersection on $x_i^\uparrow$ and $x_j^\uparrow$ (lines 6 and 7). The *Reduce* tasks collect all *keys* of *Map*'s results as candidate concepts to perform next iteration, and add the outcome to the final result (lines 8–10). When no new concepts generated, the algorithm stops and returns the set of cumulated formal concepts C.

Algorithm for Performing Big Set Operations
One criterion for the well-formedness of an ontology is that its hierarchical structure forms a lattice (Sect. 4.1). By constructing lattice graphs, we can locate those newly generated concepts in the big picture of the entire ontology and help further inspection of the concept neighbors. With lattice graphs, our result can be a used for other structure-based auditing methods, as well as for visualization.

After all formal concepts are obtained, we have a nature transitively closed relationship with respect to set inclusion. For graph rendering, we need to construct the minimal, irreducible set of subset relations as an irredundant representation of set inclusion (modular transitivity). To do so, we use distributed set operations to construct lattice graphs from the output of the concept concept construction part of MCA (Algorithm 2). We design our lattice construction algorithm by leveraging distributed big set operations using the following strategy adapted from Sects. 2.2 and 4.2. (1) get all subset relations of one concept, (2) remove other relations except for the minimal supersets. More formally, given a set X in a collection of subsets C, we use $\Uparrow X$ to denote the set of all common ancestors of X, i.e., $\Uparrow X := \{a \in C \mid \forall x \in X, x \subset a\}$. Thus, $\Uparrow X$ represents the strict upper closure of X. When X is a singleton, i.e., $X = \{x\}$, we write $\Uparrow x$ for $\Uparrow \{x\}$. Similarly, we define $\uparrow X := \{a \in C \mid \exists x \in X, x \subset a\}$. We have, for any set $X, Y \subseteq C$, $\Uparrow X = \bigcap_{a \in X} \Uparrow a$, and $\uparrow Y = \bigcup_{b \in Y} \uparrow b$. Hence, the set of minimal upper bounds of X can be obtained using the formula $\Uparrow X - \uparrow(\Uparrow X)$.

Algorithm 3: Marking Subset Relations	**Algorithm 4:** Transitivity Reduction
1 **Function** *Marking Subset Relations(C)*	1 **Function** *Transitive Reduction(CS)*
Data: Formal concept set C	**Data**: Concept-subsets pairs CS
Result: Concept-subsets pairs S	**Result**: Edge Pairs E
2 initialize HashSet $C' = Cache(C)$	2 initialize HashMap $CS' = Cache(CS)$
3 **Function** *Map(c ∈ C)*	3 **Function** *Map(cs(c, s) ∈ CS)*
4 $a = \emptyset$	4 $s' = \emptyset$
5 **foreach** $el \in C'$ **do**	5 **foreach** $el \in s$ **do**
6 **if** $el \subset c$ **then**	6 $s' \leftarrow CS'[el]$
7 $a \leftarrow el$	7 **end**
8 **end**	8 RDD< $Int, Set[Int]$ > $pair = (c, s - s')$
9 **end**	9 **Function** *Reduce(pair)*
10 RDD< $Int, Set[Int]$ > $ca = (c, a)$	10 $E \leftarrow pair$
11 **Function** *Reduce(ca(c, a))*	11 **return** E
12 $CS \leftarrow (c, a)$	12
13 **return** CS	13

The distributed big set operations involve two MapReduce jobs: *Marking Subset Relations* (Algorithm 3) and *Transitive Reduction* (Algorithm 4). The input of Algorithm 3 is the collection of all formal concepts (intents, say) obtained from Algorithm 2. First, we initialize a HashSet C' to store all concepts and distributed to all computational computers (line 2). Then, all concepts are split into partitions to perform MapReduce tasks. In each task, we collect the subsets of concept c_i by iteratively checking each element in C' to see if it is a subset of c_i (lines 3–12). The output of *Marking Subset Relations* is a collection of concept-subsets pairs (c_i, a_c), which will serve as the input of *Transitivity Reduction*. In Algorithm 4, concept and subsets pairs are first cached in CS' and sent to all nodes (line 2). Then, each *MapReduce* task removes those subsets that are the subsets of the current concept on each pair. This is achieved by removing the union of the subset list S_i for each subset i with concept c in S_c (lines 3–10).

Table 3.1 lists all the formal concepts of the formal context given in Fig. 3.3. If we equip the associated order on the concepts collection, we obtain the concept lattice shown in Fig. 3.4. In the lattice graph, C_1 contains all the intents and C_9 contains all the extents. Concepts C_1, C_2, C_3, C_4, C_5, in blue, are primitive concepts. Concepts C_7, C_8, in red, are suggested new concepts.

In Spark-MCA, each concept is represented by its intent (and refers neither to the original context, nor to any extent). One can easily incorporate a data structure for looking up the extent of a concept, after all concepts are determined. In this study, we maintain two hash maps: one is C, which, for each concept $x \in X$, collects all its attributes; similarly, the other is A, which, for each attribute $y \in Y$, collects all concepts that contain a particular attribute. Hence, the intersection $\bigcap a_i^{\downarrow}$, where a_i is the attribute of concept c_i, contains all extents of a concept. To identify the labels of formal concepts, we compare their attributes with the primitive concepts list. Concepts corresponding to the primitive concepts are naturally

Table 3.1 The list of formal concepts generated from the formal context given in Fig. 3.3

Concept	Extent	Intent
C_1	{}	{1, 2, 3, 4, 5, 6, 7, 8, 9, 10, 11, 12, 13, 14, 15, 16}
C_2	{a}	{1, 2, 3}
C_3	{b}	{4, 5, 6, 7}
C_4	{c}	{1, 2, 3, 4, 5, 6, 7, 8, 9, 10, 11}
C_5	{d}	{1, 2, 3, 4, 5, 6, 7, 12, 13, 14}
C_6	{e}	{1, 2, 3, 4, 5, 6, 7, 13, 15, 16}
C_7	{d, e}	{1, 2, 3, 4, 5, 6, 7, 13}
C_8	{c, d, e}	{1, 2, 3, 4, 5, 6, 7}
C_9	{a, b, c, d, e}	{}

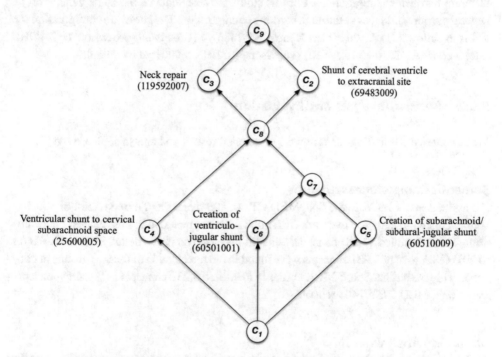

Fig. 3.4 The rendering of concepts in Table 3.1 as a lattice diagram

labeled, while the others concepts can be treated as a candidate pool of new concepts for enhancing semantic completeness.

Evaluation Method

SNOMED CT provides a "delta" file, which contains changes of concepts and relations associated with each release. To evaluate the performance of Spark-MCA, we constructed RGT by obtaining concepts that were added in the releases. Obtaining an appropriate set of changes across multiple SNOMED CT releases is not a mere job of performing unions. For the purpose of evaluation, we constructed a reference set involving two steps: (1) extract added concepts (active value: 1) from all 5 "delta" files from 201403 release to 201609 release; (2) remove deleted or revised concepts (active value: 0) from the added concept sets obtained in the first step. These remaining concepts are selected as a RGT for evaluating the result of Spark-MCA. Since the suggested concepts by Spark-MCA have no labels, we matched the corresponding concepts using their attribute sets (intents).

For scalability analysis, we executed Spark-MCA on Amazon Web Services (AWS) with different hardware configurations. For this study, we selected M4, the latest generation of general purpose instances as the main working configuration. The hardware configuration for M4 is as follows: (1) 2.3 GHz Intel Xeon® E5-2686 v4 (Broadwell) processors or 2.4 GHz Intel Xeon® E5-2676 v3 (Haswell) processors, (2) EBS-optimized by default.

3.2.2   Results, Analysis, and Evaluation

We summarize our findings as follows. For detailed results and analysis, please see [80].

Semantic Completeness Analysis

We applied Spark-MCA to the SNOMED CT 201403 release and found a total of 500,583 formal concepts suggested by Spark-MCA that were not included in this release. For evaluation, RGT identified 22,687 concepts as additions based on the 5 "delta" files from 201403 to 201609. A total of 3,231 concepts were found in the intersection of the two groups of concepts. This means that Spark-MCA correctly identified 3,231 concepts as missing concepts in the SNOMED CT 201403 release.

Scalability Analysis

Scalability is one of the hallmarks of cloud computing. We performed two scalability tests for our Spark-MCA by analyzing computational time for different subhiearchies of SNOMED CT and for different AWS configurations, respectively. For the first test, we selected 4 largest subhierarchies in SNOMED CT 201403 release: *Body structure*, *Clinical finding*, *Procedure*, and *Pharmaceutical biologic product*. We performed the test on an AWS cluster with 96 processors. The computational time for each subhierarchy is shown in Table 3.2. For the second test, we repeatedly ran Spark-MCA on the *Body structure* subhierarchy with different configurations by increasing the number of processors in the AWS cluster. We found a linear decrease of the computational time when the number of computation processors ranged from

Table 3.2 Scalability experiment on different subhierarchies in SNOMED CT

Subhierarchy	Concepts	Attributes	Time
Pharmaceutical biologic product	16,786	25,107	40 s
Body structure	30,623	45,815	3.3 mins
Clinical finding	100,652	166,123	35 mins
Procedure	54,091	99,995	93 mins

1 to 30. When the number of processors approached 100, the computational time tends to cease to decrease, indicating a threshold at which additional processors would not be helpful.

Evaluation

By comparing our results with the RGT, it was seen that 14.24% of newly added concepts can be obtained by our method. Particularly, we can see that in the 3 largest hierarchies, *Body structure*, *Clinical finding*, and *Procedure*, our Spark-MCA can identify 47.5, 18.0, and 30.2% of all newly added concepts, respectively. This indicates that Spark-MCA could be a reliable approach for addressing semantic completeness.

From Table 3.2, we can see that larger formal contexts required more computational time using our algorithm. However, we point out that because of the density and complexity, we cannot assume that a context with more objects and attributes would necessarily take more computational time (*Clinical finding* versus *Procedure*).

3.2.3   Further Discussion About the Approach and the Results

Limitation of Spark-MCA

Although our results showed Spark-MCA to be a practical method in evaluating semantic completeness, there remain a number of limitations. First, Spark-MCA cannot find those added concepts in "delta" involving newly added attributes. For example, *Difficulty swimming* (714997002) is added with a new attribute *363714003|Interprets (attribute) = 714992008|Ability to swim (observable entity)* in the 201603 release, but Spark-MCA did not include it. Other types of lexical or structure auditing methods can be useful supplements to Spark-MCA in auditing semantic completeness. Second, it is less useful to apply the FCA approach to terminological systems with very minimal semantic definitions (e.g., limited to one type of relationship).

Comparison with Related Results

We examined the example subhierarchy (hypophysectomy) provided in Jiang and Chute's work [76]. We found our results to be in agreement. However, because Jiang and Chute did not provide details about all their findings, we could not perform a more thorough comparison.

Sensitivity of the FCA-Based Model

FCA-based approach is in general known to be sensitive to the density and complexity of the input formal context. Even though Spark-MCA performed reasonably well for SNOMED CT, we did not perform similar computational experiments on other terminology systems.

Conclusion: In this section, we introduced Spark-MCA, a scalable approach for evaluating the semantic completeness of SNOMED CT using an FCA-based method on top of the Spark cloud-computing framework. We formulated SNOMED CT into a formal context in FCA and then used Spark-MCA to exhaustively compute the formal concepts of the context as well as the associated subset relations. We the applied Retrospective Ground-Truthing to assess the performance of Spark-MCA. Our results show that Spark-MCA provides a cloud-computing feasible approach for evaluating the semantic completeness of SNOMED CT using formal concept analysis.

Algorithms for Extracting Non-lattice Substructures

4

One of the desirable properties of the resulting graph structure is that the subsumption relationship (*is-a* hierarchy) should form a lattice [81]. There are in general two types of lattice-based approaches to ontology quality assurance. One involves the direct application of Formal Concept Analysis (FCA [82]), mostly for auditing semantic completeness or missing concepts [76]. The second involves the extraction of lattice-violating fragments (discussed in Sects. 4.1 and 4.2), or *non-lattice fragments* (note that *non-lattice fragments* and *non-lattice subgraphs* are used interchangeably in this book), which represent violations of the FCA principle that systematic engineering approaches for constructing concept hierarchies always result in order structures that are lattices in the sense of lattice theory [82]. This non-lattice approach for ontology quality assurance involves the extraction of graph substructures (i.e., sub-orders) that violate the *lattice property*, which states that any two concept nodes have at most one minimal shared (common) ancestor and at most one maximal shared descendant.

The use of the non-lattice approach for improving the quality of an ontology consists of the following general steps:

1. Identify node-pairs that violate the lattice property (i.e., non-lattice pairs) and extract the associated non-lattice fragments;
2. Detect ontological defects such as miss-aligned is-a relations or missing concepts in the extracted non-lattice fragments, often leveraging additional or external information;
3. Formulate and generate change suggestions automatically and present the suggestions in a usable format;
4. Perform reviews of the suggested changes and accepts or rejects such suggestions by a qualified ontology engineer or ontology editor, and incorporate the accepted changes into the next release.

As discussed in Sect. 5.2 the non-lattice approach is unique in that while most ontology quality assurance techniques [28] merely identify potential errors, this approach can not

© The Author(s), under exclusive license to Springer Nature Switzerland AG 2022 73
G.-Q. Zhang et al., *Formal Methods for the Analysis of Biomedical Ontologies*,
Synthesis Lectures on Data, Semantics, and Knowledge,
https://doi.org/10.1007/978-3-031-12131-9_4

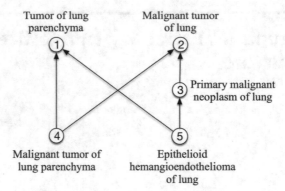

(A) Non-lattice fragment in SNOMED CT

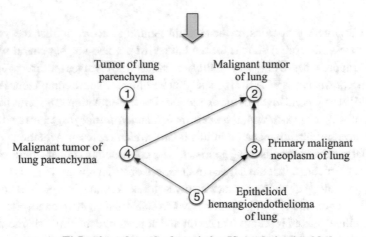

(B) Lattice subgraph after missing IS-A relation is added

Fig. 4.1 An example **A** of non-lattice fragment of size 5 in SNOMED CT, as well as the resulting lattice subgraph **B** after a missing *is-a* relation is added (red link)

only identify previously undiscovered errors confirmed by domain experts, but also suggest appropriate remediation (i.e., "auto-suggestion"). For example, Fig. 4.1, extracted from the September 2017 release of SNOMED CT (US edition), contains a substructure (A) of *is-a* relations on the left, involving 5 concepts. This is a non-lattice fragment, because the concept nodes labeled 1 and 2 have two maximal shared descendants: concept nodes labeled 4 and 5.

With a combination of structural and lexical information represented in this fragment, one can infer that "*Epithelioid hemangioendothelioma of lung*" *is-a* "*Malignant tumor of lung parenchyma*." Remarkably, adding such a missing edge (in red color) also makes the resulting subgraph (1B) conforming to the lattice property: concept nodes labeled 1 and 2 now have a unique maximal shared descendant: concept nodes labeled 4 (since concept 5

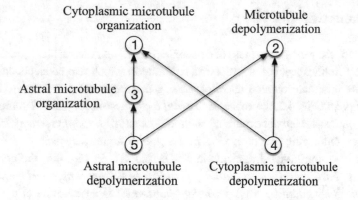

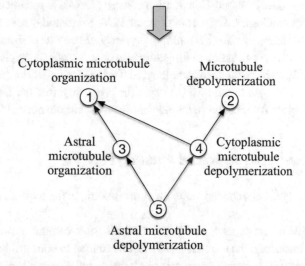

(B) Lattice subgraph after missing IS-A relation is added

Fig. 4.2 An example **A** of non-lattice fragment of size 5 in the Gene Ontology, as well as the resulting lattice subgraph **B** after a missing *is-a* relation is added (red link)

is no longer "maximal"). Similarly, Fig. 4.2 shows a non-lattice fragment (A) in the Gene Ontology (GO) on the left, and the corrected structure (B) on the right.

Both the FCA- and the non-lattice-based approaches incur computational costs that sometimes make exhaustive analyses prohibitive, and therefore, scalable algorithms need to be developed to address this computational challenge.

4.1   Exhaustive Analysis

One criterion for the well-formedness of ontologies is that their hierarchical structure forms a lattice [81]. Simply speaking, a lattice is a structure in which two concepts do not share more than one minimal common ancestor. Lattice fragments are pervasive in SNOMED CT. For example, in Fig. 4.3, the concepts "*Partial hypophysectomy*" and "*Transsphenoidal hypophysectomy*" share only one minimal common ancestor, "*Hypophysectomy*." This illustrates a lattice-conforming structure, a.k.a. *lattice pair* or *lattice fragment*.

There are also non-lattice fragments in SNOMED CT. In Fig. 4.4, the concept pair (colored blue) "*Partial excision of pituitary gland by transfrontal approach*" and "*Partial excision of pituitary gland by transsphenoidal approach*" is an example of a *non-lattice pair*, because this pair shares more than one minimal common ancestor (namely "*Partial hypophysectomy*" and "*Transcranial hypophysectomy*," colored red).

We introduce **La**ttice-based **S**tructural **A**uditing (*LaSA*), a methodology for auditing large biomedical ontologies. *LaSA* complements FCA-based and other existing approaches to ontological auditing by *taking the lattice-property directly as a structural principle for ontologies*. The main contribution of this study is to demonstrate the applicability of *LaSA* to the entirety of a large biomedical terminology: SNOMED CT (>300 k concepts). Our results are consistent with those based on FCA, with the advantage that the *LaSA* computational pipeline is scalable and applicable to ontological systems without normal form presentations.

4.1.1   Lattice-Based Structural Auditing Pipeline

LaSA exhaustively checks concept pairs for conformation to the requirement of being a part of a lattice.

For each pair of concepts *a* and *b*, we find all their common ancestors. Among all their common ancestors, the minimal ones must be unique to conform to the mathematical definition of a lattice, in which every pair of elements must have a (unique) *least common ancestor*.

Fig. 4.3 A lattice fragment in SNOMED CT's *Hypophysectomy* sub-hierarchy in Procedures. The blue nodes share a unique minimal common ancestor

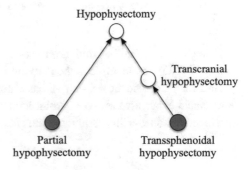

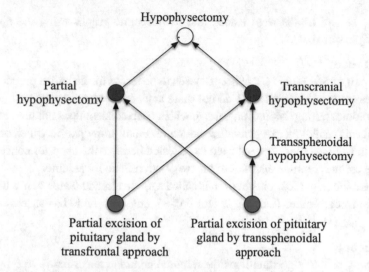

Fig. 4.4 A non-lattice fragment in SNOMED CT's *Hypophysectomy* sub-hierarchy. The red nodes share more than one minimal common ancestor

Our method for identifying non-lattice fragments involves three steps: (1) acquiring SNOMED CT data; (2) selecting probes; (3) testing probes.

Acquiring SNOMED CT Data

From the distribution of SNOMED CT, we extracted all the *is-a* relations among active concepts. We created URIs for all SNOMED CT concepts and *used the rdfs:subClassOf predicate to represent the is-a relation*. Then we computed the transitive closure of the *is-a* relation and created a distinct set of triples for it.

Algorithm 1: Finding minimal common ancestors

> **Data:** Transitively closed RDF-triple store and probe
> (a, b)
> **Output:** The minimal common ancestors of a, b
> **1** Set *count* to 0 for each node;
> **2 if** *?sb is a common ancestor of a, b* **then**
> **3** | increment *count*(*?sb*) by 1
> **4 end**
> **5 if** *?sb is an ancestor of a common ancestor ?sa of a, b*
>   **then**
> **6** | increment *count*(*?sb*) by 1
> **7 end**
> **8** Sort *?sb* in ascending order according to its *count*;
> **9** Mark all *?sb* with *count*(*?sb*) = 1 as minimal common
>   ancestor

The two sets of triples were loaded into two separate graphs using the open source Virtuoso triple store [61].

Selecting Probes

Not every pair of SNOMED CT concepts needs to be tested for its lattice properties. Since the 19 hierarchies in SNOMED CT do not share any concepts, only pairs within the same hierarchy require testing. Moreover, pairs in which each concept does not have at least two parent concepts cannot form a non-lattice structure. Finally, any pair in which one concept is an ancestor of the other does not need to be tested because the ancestor concept in such pairs is the unique common ancestor of the two, with reflexivity assumed.

More formally, a pair of concepts a, b is called a *probe* if a and b are not in a hierarchical relationship to each other (i.e., $a \not\sqsubseteq b$ and $b \not\sqsubseteq a$), and each node has at least two direct parents.

Testing Probes

The following simple algorithm finds the minimal common ancestors of a, b by counting the instances of two specific cases where a node is situated as a part of the common ancestor subgraph. The key insight, however, is the idea of keeping track of appropriate counts.

To implement Algorithm 9, we construct a two-part SPARQL query executed against a transitively-closed graph of *is-a* relations.

The first part of the query (Fig. 4.5) finds all common ancestors and tracks the result by having each common ancestor receive 1 as the *counts*.

This is straightforward using the SPARQL query

$$a \text{ rdfs:subClassOf } ?sb$$
$$b \text{ rdfs:subClassOf } ?sb$$

to get hold of all nodes $?sb$ that are ancestors of a and b.

The second part of the query (Fig. 4.6) finds all common ancestors that are *ancestors among the common ancestors* – those nodes $?sb$ that are above a common ancestor $?sa$. This can be achieved by the SPARQL query

$$a \quad \text{rdfs:subClassOf } ?sa$$
$$b \quad \text{rdfs:subClassOf } ?sa$$
$$?sa \text{ rdfs:subClassOf } ?sb$$

The counts for $?sb$ here keep track of the in-degrees of each node in the common-ancestor subgraph.

From the union of the two parts of the query, nodes x and y receive a total count of 1, respectively; they are the minimal common ancestors of a and b.

LaSA separates two kinds of probes: those with a unique minimal common ancestor, and those with more than one minimal common ancestor. The latter is an indication of a non-lattice fragment.

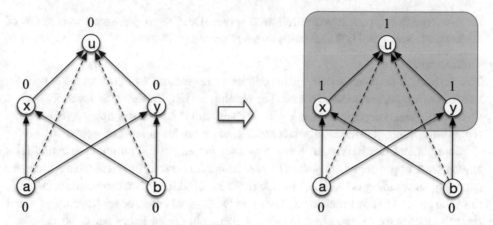

Fig. 4.5 SPARQL query finding all common ancestors of a, b, with each such ancestor receiving count 1. Dashed edges represent those due to the effect of transitive closure

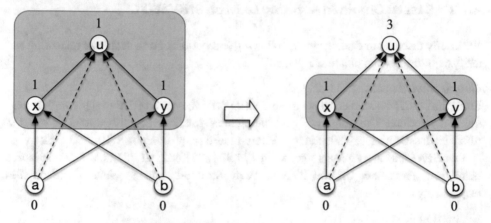

Fig. 4.6 SPARQL query finding all common ancestors of a, b, with each such ancestor receiving count 1 if it is above some other such ancestor

Implementation

The algorithms presented earlier for selecting the probes to be tested, and testing them, were implemented without any ad hoc programming. Generic queries were created for each algorithm and subpart thereof and loaded as stored procedures. We used a simple script to compute the cartesian product of all pairs of concepts within a given hierarchy of SNOMED CT. Through this script, each pair was evaluated as a potential probe (by querying a stored procedure instantiated with the pair). If qualified as a probe, the pair was then tested for its lattice properties by querying a second stored procedure. The results were stored in text files for further processing. The open source Virtuoso RDF store version 06.00.3123 was used for this experiment, running on a Dell 2950 server (Dual Xeon processor) with 32 GB of memory. A total of 500,000 9kB buffers were allocated to Virtuoso.

Optimization

This subsection describes a strategy that checks for the existence of greatest lower bounds, rather than least upper bounds, achieved by running SPARQL queries "in reverse."

On average, concepts in ontological hierarchies tend to have fewer upper-level concepts representing more general and abstract entities, and more lower level concepts.

Since lattices can be viewed either top-down or bottom-up, only one direction (i.e., among least upper bounds or greatest lower bounds) needs to be tested. Since there are generally more concepts lower in a hierarchy (as in SNOMED CT's taxonomic backbone), this motivates us to test for maximal bounds in the original order, or equivalently, minimal upper bounds in the reverse order, to reduce the number of non-lattice pairs.

4.1.2   Results Obtained Applying LaSA on SNOMED CT

We briefly discuss our findings in the following subsections. For a detailed explanation and analysis of the results, please see [83, 84].

Quantitative Results

From the 307,754 active concepts in SNOMED CT, we created RDF triples for representing *is-a* relations. The graph of direct hierarchical relations contains a total of 439,733 rdfs:subClassOf triples, while the transitively-closed graph contains 1,191,796 triples.

Our SPARQL query results uncovered 174,574; 251,662; 91,787; and 889 non-lattice pairs from Procedure, Clinical Finding, Body Structure, and Specimen subhierarchies respectively.

Evaluation

We ran our *LaSA* algorithm on the Hypophysectomy sub-hierarchy of SNOMED CT, the running example included in Jiang and Chute [76], using the same version of SNOMED CT as was used in their study, and performed a systematic comparison of our respective results.

In FCA, anonymous nodes correspond to missing concepts combining several properties (e.g., hypophysectomy + transfrontal approach). Jiang and Chute found five anonymous nodes using FCA; we also found exactly five non-lattice pairs. Three non-lattice pairs correspond exactly to the three anonymous nodes (1, 3, and 4 in Table 3, page 95 of [76]), with a perfect match between our non-lattice pair and the extensions constructed using FCA.

The two remaining non-lattice pairs are part of the extension for Node 5. However, we found no non-lattice counterpart for Node 2. Upon closer inspection, the extension of Node 2 in Jiang and Chute represents a case of an anonymous node without any lattice-violation. The creation of the intermediary node "*Transfrontal hypophysectomy*" would be justified only because several subtypes of excision of the pituitary gland by transfrontal approach are described, not to create a unique lowest common ancestor for these subtypes of hypophysectomy. Our findings are therefore consistent with that of Jiang and Chute, but FCA identified one anonymous node, which *LaSA* cannot identify.

4.1.3   Precoordination and the Lattice Property

There is a close relation between precoordination and the lattice properties of the terminology. Two sibling concepts denoting multiple features (including two common features) will form a lattice only if their lowest common ancestor represents both features (and will not form a lattice if each common feature is represented by a distinct ancestor). As can be seen from Fig. 4.7, the concepts colored in blue *"Tissue specimen from breast"* and *"Tissue specimen from heart"* share the features of being a kind of tissue specimen and a kind of specimen from trunk. In SNOMED CT, this is represented by two edges shared by the two blue concepts to *"Tissue specimen"* and to *"Specimen from trunk,"* which is the reason why this fragment is not a lattice. In order to transform this fragment into a lattice, a new concept *"Tissue specimen from trunk"* would need to be created, which would be the direct descendant of the current minimal common ancestors and would become a new unique lowest common ancestor of *"Tissue specimen from breast"* and *"Tissue specimen from heart."*

Beyond the technicalities (i.e., the structural properties of the terminology), one question for SNOMED CT is how much precoordination is needed in clinical applications. The concept *"Tissue specimen from trunk"* is a valid concept, but it is unclear whether such intermediary nodes would be useful to users. (*"Tissue specimen from mediastinum"* would be a legitimate candidate as well). On the one hand, having many precoordinated terms would reduce the need for having to deal with post-coordination, which is nontrivial for most users. On the other, tens of thousands of such precoordinated nodes are likely to be needed to transform SNOMED CT into a lattice, which comes at a cost in terms of maintenance (for the developers) and in terms of increased volume for the users.

Fig. 4.7 Non-lattice pair from the Specimen hierarchy

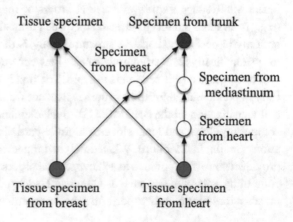

From a quality assurance perspective [28], what is important is to ensure that precoordination is used consistently in SNOMED CT, so as to facilitate usage. This, for example, would be an argument in favor of the creation of a concept *"Transfrontal hypophysectomy,"* as suggested by Jiang and Chute, in order to mirror, e.g., *"Transsphenoidal hypophysectomy."* More generally, however, one limitation of our approach is that it is not sufficient to determine automatically whether non-lattice fragments correspond to errors (i.e., whether the missing concepts identified are clinically relevant).

Conclusion: *LaSA* produces results consistent with the FCA-based approach of Jiang & Chute, without suffering from their computational scalability problem. Additionally, unlike FCA, *LaSA* is applicable to ontological systems consisting mostly of taxonomic links, without requiring a normal formal presentation. Among the methods developed for quality assurance in SNOMED CT, *LaSA* has been effective in identifying (potentially) missing precoordinated concepts in SNOMED CT. A model of desirable (vs. excessive) precoordination should be developed, which could be used in conjunction with *LaSA* in order to determine which lattice violations are indicative of problems and require the attention of the editors of the terminology system. Meanwhile, we have shown that a lattice-based approach is applicable to large-scale terminologies and can be implemented with minimal programming effort.

4.2   Ontologies as Big Knowledge Graph Data

This section presents progresses made in using a scalable cloud computing environment, Hadoop and MapReduce [85], to perform ontology quality assurance (OQA), and points to areas of future opportunity. The standard sequential approach used for implementing OQA methods can take weeks, if not months, for exhaustive analyses for large biomedical ontological systems. With OQA methods newly implemented using massively parallel algorithms in the MapReduce framework, several orders of magnitude in speed-up can be achieved (e.g., from three months to three hours). Such dramatically reduced time makes it feasible not only to perform exhaustive structural analysis of large ontological hierarchies but also to systematically track structural changes between versions for evolutional analysis.

The purpose of this section is twofold. The first is to introduce key elements in successfully implementing algorithms in the MapReduce framework to perform evolutional analysis and visualization on the SNOMED CT. Such elements include MapReduce algorithms for computing global and local closures in finite partially ordered sets, and for large set operations (union, intersection). When combined together, the closures and set operations can provide a powerful approach to achieve several orders of magnitude in speed-up using cloud computing environments such as Cloudera Hadoop. Such dramatically reduced time then makes it feasible not only to perform exhaustive structural analysis of large ontological hierarchies, but also to systematically track structural changes between versions for evolutional analysis.

The second purpose of this section is to describe opportunities in three areas in using a Big Data approach for OQA: one is to extend the scope of the MapReduce-based approach to existing OQA methods, especially for automated exhaustive structural analysis. The second is to apply our MaPLE pipeline, demonstrated as an exemplar method for SNOMED CT, to other biomedical ontologies. The third area is to develop interfaces for reviewing results obtained by OQA methods and for visualizing ontological alignment and evolution, which can also take advantage of cloud computing technology to systematically pre-compute computationally intensive jobs in order to increase performance during user interactions with the visualization interface. Progress in these directions is expected to better support the ontological engineering lifecycle.

4.2.1 Big Data Approach

Here, we introduce our Big Data approach MaPLE to performing lattice-based OQA. Figure 4.8 shows an overview of the MaPLE pipeline. It takes a partially ordered set (poset) as input, computing global closure and local closures (a key step to facilitate parallel exhaustive analysis), and detects all non-lattice pairs and relation reversals, which are stored in a database for a web-based interface to visualize evolutional structural changes.

Theoretical Background for Computing Minimal Upper Bounds

MaPLE takes a partially ordered set (poset) as input and generates the collection of all non-lattice pairs in the poset. For example, in the poset given in Fig. 1.5 (right), we have $\text{mub}\{1, 2\} = \{6, 7\}$, so the size of $\text{mub}\{1, 2\}$ is 2, making $(1, 2)$ a non-lattice pair in this poset. On the other hand, we have $\text{mub}\{1, 3\} = \{7\}$, and so $(1, 3)$ is a lattice pair. Thus, finding non-lattice pairs requires computing the minimal upper bounds for each candidate pair, achieved through a sequence of set-theoretic operations using closures as explained next.

Given a set X of elements in a poset L, we use $\Uparrow X$ to denote the set of all common ancestors of X, i.e., $\Uparrow X := \{a \mid \forall x \in X, x < a\}$, where $x < a$ means $x \leq a$ but $x \neq a$.

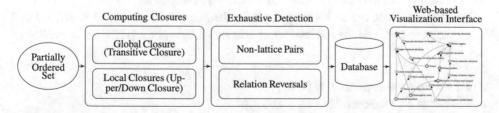

Fig. 4.8 An overview of the MaPLE pipeline

Note that $X \cap (\Uparrow X)$ is always empty. When X is a singleton, i.e., $X = \{x\}$, we write $\Uparrow x$ for $\Uparrow\{x\}$. Similarly, we define $\uparrow X := \{a \mid \exists x \in X, x < a\}$. Thus, $\uparrow X$ represents its strict upper closure. Dually, its strict down closure $\downarrow X$ is defined as $\downarrow X := \{a \mid \exists x \in X, a < x\}$. In the followings, we refer upper closure and down closure of X to its strict upper closure and down closure respectively. It is straightforward to check that for any set $X, Y \subseteq L$,

$$\Uparrow X = \bigcap_{a \in X} \Uparrow a, \quad \text{and} \quad \uparrow Y = \bigcup_{b \in Y} \uparrow b.$$

For singletons, we have $\Uparrow x = \uparrow x$. Two elements x, y are called *incomparable* if neither $x \leq y$, nor $y \leq x$.

Before we introduce Theorem 4.2 for computing minimal upper bounds, the following lemma should be helpful (whose proof is omitted):

Lemma 4.1 *Let x, y be elements in a poset L. If $y \leq x$ but $x \notin \uparrow y$, then $x = y$.*

Theorem 4.2 *Let X be a set of pairwise incomparable elements of a poset L, with the size of X at least two. We have*

$$\text{mub}(X) = \Uparrow X - \uparrow(\Uparrow X).$$

Proof Let $m \in \Uparrow X - \uparrow(\Uparrow X)$. Since $m \in \Uparrow X$, m is an upper bound of X. Since $m \notin \uparrow(\Uparrow X)$, we have $m \notin \uparrow t$ for each $t \in \Uparrow X$. For any upper bound u of X (i.e., $x \leq u$ for each $x \in X$) with $u \leq m$, we need to show that $u = m$. Since u is an upper bound of X, which contains at least two incomparable elements, we have $u \in \Uparrow X$. Also, because $m \notin \uparrow t$ for each $t \in \Uparrow X$, we have $m \notin \uparrow u$. By Lemma 4.1, $m = u$. Hence, m is a minimal upper bound of X. □

A special case for Theorem 4.2 is a pair of incomparable elements x and y, which is stated as:

$$\text{mub}(\{x, y\}) = (\uparrow x \cap \uparrow y) - \bigcup_{t \in \uparrow x \cap \uparrow y} \uparrow t. \qquad (4.1)$$

It is worth noting that computing minimal upper bound using upper closures enables the massive parallel processing implemented in MapReduce framework, without worrying about the dependencies among steps in traditional sequential algorithms.

We illustrate these results by an example. In the poset shown in Fig. 4.9, nodes 1 and 2 are incomparable, and the minimal upper bounds of them, $\text{mub}\{1, 2\}$, are calculated as follows:

- Find node 1's ancestors: $\uparrow 1 = \{4, 6, 7, 8\}$;
- Find node 2's ancestors: $\uparrow 2 = \{3, 5, 6, 7, 8\}$;
- Perform intersection: $\uparrow 1 \cap \uparrow 2 = \{6, 7, 8\}$, which gives common ancestors of 1 and 2;
- Evaluate $\bigcup_{t \in \uparrow 1 \cap \uparrow 2} \uparrow t : \uparrow 6 \cup \uparrow 7 \cup \uparrow 8 = \{8\} \cup \{8\} \cup \emptyset = \{8\}$;
- Compute set difference: $\uparrow 1 \cap \uparrow 2 - \bigcup_{t \in \uparrow 1 \cap \uparrow 2} \uparrow t = \{6, 7\}$.

Fig. 4.9 A simple poset used to illustrate the order-theoretic notions

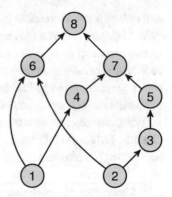

By Theorem 4.2, $\text{mub}\{1, 2\} = \{6, 7\}$, which is precisely what we need. Therefore, $(1, 2)$ is a non-lattice pair in the poset given in Fig. 4.9.

MapReduce for Computing Closures

Algorithm 2: MapReduce Algorithm for Computing Transitive Closure Pairs

Input: Concepts and *is-a* relation pairs of concepts
     `/* c₁ is-a c₂ means c₂ is a direct parent of c₁ */`
Output: Transitive closure pairs
1 Initialization: setup a HashMap CP and load it with concepts and their direct parents using *DistributedCache*
2 *Map (concept c)*
3     $P = CP\text{.get}(c)$ `/* Get direct parents of c */`
4     $A = \emptyset$ `/* Initialize a set for ancestors of c */`
5   **while** $P \neq \emptyset$ **do**
6        $A\text{.add}(P)$
7        $temp = \emptyset$
8   **for** *each concept p in P* **do**
9           $temp\text{.add}(CP\text{.get}(p))$
10   **end**
11       $P = temp$
12   **end**
13   Emit (c, A)
14 **end**
15 *Reduce (concept c, concept ancestors A)*
16   **for** *each concept a in A* **do**
17   Emit (c, a) `/* Output transitive closure pairs */`
18   **end**
19 **end**

In this subsection, we present MapReduce algorithms for computing global transitive closure pairs, and local upper-closures and down-closures. Algorithm 2 shows the initialization, map and reduce steps to compute transitive closure pairs given a set of concepts and *is-a* relation pairs of concepts (poset), where c_1 *is-a* c_2 means c_2 is a direct parent of c_1. First, a hash map of concepts and their direct parents is loaded by all the mappers. Then in the map phase, each mapper reads in a concept and recursively collects its ancestors, level by level, until no direct parents can be found. In the reduce phase, each reducer emits the concept-ancestor pairs for each concept it processes.

Based on the computed transitive closure pairs, upper-closures (Algorithm 3), and down-closures (Algorithm 4) are also calculated using MapReduce resulting in a collection of concept-upper-closure pairs $(c, {\uparrow}c)$ and concept-down-closure pairs $(c, {\downarrow}c)$.

Algorithm 3: MapReduce Algorithm for Computing Upper-closures

Input: Transitive closure pairs
Output: Concept upper-closures

1
2 *Map (concept c, ancestor a)*
3   Emit (c, a)
4 **end**
5
6 *Reduce (concept c, upper-closure $\{a_1, a_2, \ldots\}$)*
7   Emit $(c, \{a_1, a_2, \ldots\})$ /* Output concept c and its upper-closure */
8 **end**

Given a set of transitive closure pairs of concepts, the MapReduce program described in Algorithm 3 simply collects upper-closure for each concept. In the map phase, each mapper reads in a set of transitively closed concept pairs and emits key-value pairs (c, a) where c is a concept and a is an ancestor of c. In the reduce phase, each reducer collects the upper-closure ${\uparrow}c = \{a_1, a_2, \ldots\}$ of a concept c and emits concept-upper-closure pairs $(c, {\uparrow}c)$. Similarly, Algorithm 4 collects down-closure for each concept by reversing the order of the input transitive closure pairs.

Algorithm 4: MapReduce Algorithm for Computing Down-closures

Input: Transitive closure pairs
Output: Concept down-closures

1
2 *Map (concept c, ancestor a)*
3   Emit (a, c) /* Reverse the order of the input pair */
4 **end**
5
6 *Reduce (concept a, down-closure $\{c_1, c_2, \ldots\}$)*
7   Emit $(a, \{c_1, c_2, \ldots\})$ /* Output concept a and its down-closure */
8 **end**

The upper-closures obtained in Algorithm 3 and down-closures obtained in Algorithm 4 will be used for detecting non-lattice pairs in Sect. 4.2.1 and generating ontological fragments.

MapReduce for Computing Non-lattice Pairs
Algorithm 5 shows the MapReduce algorithm for detecting non-lattice pairs. The input is the pre-computed concept-upper-closure pairs $(c, \uparrow c)$. In implementation, such input concept-upper-closure pairs are not only split and fed into multiple mappers, but also read by all the mappers and reducers as *DistributedCache* in Hadoop and stored in a hash map called CA. In the map stage, each mapper generates candidate pairs for each concept c_1 by iterating through each concept c_2 in CA, checking if c_1's concept identifier is less than c_2's concept identifier to ensure the uniqueness of the pair. A concept pair (c_1, c_2) is then emitted as a key and their upper-closures $(\uparrow c_1, \uparrow c_2)$ where $\uparrow c_1 = \{a_{11}, a_{12}, \ldots\}$, $\uparrow c_2 = \{a_{21}, a_{22}, \ldots\}$, respectively, as a value. The requirement that c_1's concept identifier is less than c_2's concept identifier avoids the situation that the same concept pair generates two different keys. In the reduce stage, each reducer checks if c_1 and c_2 in a concept pair are incomparable, calculates their minimal upper bounds, and emits pairs with more than one minimal upper bound as keys and their minimal upper bounds as values.

Optimization Strategies To reduce the total number of input and resulting pairs yet without missing any non-lattice fragments, we incorporate two optimization strategies in MaPLE implementation, which are discussed in Sect. 4.1.

• Leveraging Duality and Reversing Order.
  After obtaining the transitive closure of a set of SNOMED CT pairs $\{(c, a)\}$, we reverse the pairs and take the pairs $\{(a, c)\}$ as input for MaPLE. Ontological hierarchies have a "fan-out" shape: they tend to have fewer upper-level concepts representing more general entities while having lower level concepts representing more specific entities. For example, for the poset in Fig. 4.10, the upward direction has 10 non-lattice pairs: for each distinct $a, b \in \{1, 2, 3, 4, 5\}$, we have mub$(\{a, b\}) = \{6.7\}$. However, in the downward

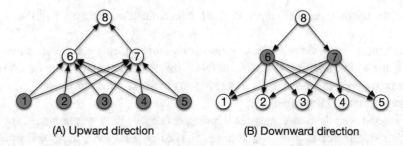

(A) Upward direction   (B) Downward direction

Fig. 4.10 Illustrative example showing a smaller number of non-lattice pairs in the reverse (downward) direction (**B**) as oppose to upward direction (**A**)

Algorithm 5: MapReduce Algorithm for Computing Non-lattice Pairs

---

Input: Concept-upper-closure pairs

Output: Non-lattice pairs and their minimal upper bounds

1 ;

2 Initialization: setup a HashMap CA and load it with concept and its upper-closure using
   DistributedCache;

3 ;

4 *Map* $(c_1, \{a_{11}, a_{12}, \ldots\})$

5   **for** *each concept* c_2 *in* CA **do**

6   **if** $c_1.\text{ID} < c_2.\text{ID}$ **then**

7   Emit $((c_1, c_2), (\{a_{11}, a_{12}, \ldots\}, \{a_{21}, a_{22}, \ldots\}))$;   /* Generate candidate
            pairs */

8   **end**

9   **end**

10 **end**

11 ;

12 *Reduce* $((c_1, c_2), \{(\{a_{11}, a_{12}, \ldots\}, \{a_{21}, a_{22}, \ldots\})\})$

13    $N \leftarrow \{a_{11}, a_{12}, \ldots\} \cup \{a_{21}, a_{22}, \ldots\}$;   /* Union c_1's and c_2's
      upper-closures */

14   **if** $c_1 \notin N$ *and* $c_2 \notin N$ **then**   /* If c_1 and c_2 are incomparable */

15       $A \leftarrow \{a_{11}, a_{12}, \ldots\} \cap \{a_{21}, a_{22}, \ldots\}$;   /* Intersect c_1's and c_2's
      upper-closures */

16       $U \leftarrow \emptyset$;

17   **for** *each concept* a *in* A **do**

18          $U \leftarrow U \cup CA.\text{get}(a)$;   /* Union a's upper-closures */

19   **end**

20       $B \leftarrow A - U$;   /* Calculate minimal upper bounds */

21   **if** $|B| > 1$ **then**

22   Emit$((c_1, c_2), B)$;   /* Output non-lattice pairs */

23   **end**

24   **end**

25 **end**

---

direction, the only non-lattice pair is $\{6, 7\}$, confirming the observation of the "fan-out"
effect.

Since lattices can be viewed either top-down or bottom-up, only one direction needs to be
tested for lattice property. The effect of this is that instead of computing minimal upper
bounds, we compute the maximal lower bounds in the original hierarchy.

- Concepts with a Unique Parent.

The second optimization strategy is skipping concepts with a unique parent (or dually,
children) in the map stage of Algorithm 5. The rationale for considering concepts with a
single parent is that whenever such a concept is involved in a non-lattice pair, there must
be an ancestor of this concept already involved in a non-lattice fragment.

MapReduce Algorithm for Computing Non-lattice Fragments

The non-lattice fragment around an input non-lattice pair is a subgraph consisting of all the concept nodes between any of the non-lattice pair and any of the maximal common lower bounds.

Algorithm 6: MapReduce Algorithm for Computing Non-lattice Fragments

Input: Non-lattice pairs and their maximal lower bounds as well as concept upper-closures and down-closures

Output: Non-lattice fragments

1

2 Initialization: setup two hash maps CU and CD and load them with concept upper-closures and down-closures using *DistributedCache*, respectively

3

4 *Map (non-lattice pair C, maximal lower bounds L)*

5      $U \leftarrow C \cup L$ /* Initialize U with C and L */

6   **for** *each concept c in C* **do**

7   **for** *each concept l in L* **do**

8              $U \leftarrow U \cup (CD.\text{get}(c) \cap CU.\text{get}(l))$ /* Union $\downarrow c \cap \uparrow l$ */

9   **end**

10   **end**

11   Emit (C, U)

12 **end**

We use non-lattice pairs and their maximal lower bounds as seed concepts to generate the corresponding non-lattice fragments. Given a non-lattice pair of concepts $C = \{c_1, c_2\}$ and the set L of their maximal lower bounds, the corresponding non-lattice fragment is computed as follows:

$$C \cup L \cup \bigcup_{c \in C, l \in L} \{\downarrow c \cap \uparrow l\} \qquad (4.2)$$

Algorithm 6 shows the MapReduce algorithm to compute non-lattice fragments. First two hash maps are built to store concepts and their upper-closures and down-closures, and distribute them to every computing nodes. Then, in the map phase, each mapper reads in a non-lattice pair of concepts C and their maximal lower bounds L, finds down-closures for the concepts in C and upper-closures for the concepts in L from the hash maps, and performs set operations to get the non-lattice fragment. The non-lattice pairs and their corresponding non-lattice fragments are emitted. Note that there is no reduce phase since the map phase outputs the desired result.

Complexity Analysis

We analyze the time complexity of the presented MapReduce algorithms as follows. Note that when there is any loop involved, we used the maximum number of possible iterations needed as the worst case to estimate the computation time.

1. Time complexity for MapReduce computation of transitive closures (Algorithm 2). Let N be the number of concept nodes, d be the maximum depth of the ontological graph, m be the number of Mappers, and r be the number of Reducers. The time complexity for the map phase of Algorithm 2 is estimated to be $O(d \times p \times N/m)$, where p is the maximum number of direct parents of concepts. The reason for this is that for each node, the algorithm iteratively collects all direct parents from the current set of concepts. The time complexity for the reduce phase of Algorithm 2 is $O(a \times N/r)$, where a is the maximum number of ancestors of concepts.

2. Time complexity for MapReduce computation of upper- and down-closures (Algorithms 3 and 4). The map phrase takes $O(N/m)$, and the reduce phase takes $O(N/r)$, where N is the size of pairs in the transitive closure, m is the number of Mappers, and r is the number of Reducers. Note that the overall transitive closure is the input, so no recursive inspection of node neighborhood is required. This is the most suitable task for MapReduce: shuffling.

3. Time complexity for MapReduce computation for detecting non-lattice pairs (Algorithm 5). One basic step for Algorithm 4 is to compute a Cartesian product (all possible pairs of concepts and their local closures). There are different ways one can compute Cartesian product depending on the RAM sizes of compute nodes; we use a simple approach by keeping a copy as the MapReduce input, and the second copy as cache distributed to all compute nodes (which should be able to store an entire copy of N concepts and local closures in the RAM). The time complexity is $O(N^2/m)$ for the map phase and $O(c \times N^2/r)$ for the reduce phase, where m is the number of Mappers, r is the number of Reducers, and c is the factor accounting for the time needed to perform set intersection and union operations in the reduce phase.

4. Time complexity for MapReduce computation for computing non-lattice fragments (Algorithm 6). Let N be the number of non-lattice pairs, l be the largest number of maximal lower bounds for non-lattice pairs, and m be the number of Mappers. Then the time complexity to compute non-lattice fragments is $O(c \times l \times N/m)$, where c is the factor accounting for time needed to perform set intersection and union operations.

In the above analysis of time complexity, we did not investigate the load balancing problem of the MapReduce algorithms, which could potentially further improve the computational efficiency. In addition, we omitted the time needed for setting up and preloading cache in certain algorithms, since they will be linearly proportional to the input size and performed only once per each run of the algorithm.

4.2.2 Experiment Results

The following subsections contain a summary of the results. For detailed analysis and discussion of results, please see [86, 87].

Experimental Hadoop Environment
All the MapReduce algorithms implemented in this section were run on a private cloud using Cloudera Hadoop 4.3 (Hadoop 2.0.0-cdh4.3.0) with 1 master node and 30 slave nodes. The master node uses a dual quad-core Intel Xeon 5150 2.66 GHz, while the compute nodes are machines with dual quad-core Intel Xeon 5450 3.0 GHz processors, all running RedHat Enterprise Linux 6.4. Each node has a local 146 GB SAS hard drive. Each server has 16 GB of RAM. The compute nodes are interconnected using a low-latency 10 Gigabit Ethernet network based on Arista switches and Intel NetEffects Ethernet adapters.

Basic SNOMED CT Statistics and Non-lattice Pairs
Running MaPLE on 07/2009 version of SNOMED CT containing a total of 306,627 concepts and 445,549 *is-a* relations, we obtained 559,182 non-lattice pairs in 10,168 seconds. Meanwhile running MaPLE on 03/2014 version containing 299,286 concepts and 445,357 relations resulted in 586,771 non-lattice pairs in 11,166 seconds.

Changes on Non-lattice Pairs During SNOMED CT Evolution
With dramatically reduced time for analysis, 3 hours instead of 3 months, MaPLE allows us to track the changes of non-lattice pairs between different versions. Figure 4.11 shows the summary of the differences between SNOMED CT versions using the percentage of non-lattice pair changes. We use $|N - O|/|N|$ and $|O - N|/|O|$ to show the difference. Here $|X|$ stands for the size of the set X. Therefore, $|N - O|/|N|$ is the percentage of non-lattice pairs which are newly added to the later version. $|O - N|/|O|$ is the percentage of non-lattice pairs which are removed from the previous version. It is important to note that

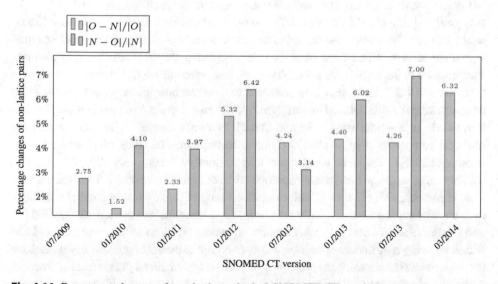

Fig. 4.11 Percentage changes of non-lattice pairs in 8 SNOMED CT versions

$|N - O| \neq |N| - |O|$ in general – we can have two equal-sized sets that have nothing in common, and so in the extreme, $|N - O| = |N|$ but $|N| - |O| = 0$.

The colored bars in Fig. 4.11 show the percentage changes between versions of SNOMED CT. Comparing the 01/2010 version with the 07/2009 version, we found 15,582 non-lattice pairs in the 01/2010 version but not in the 07/2009 version ($N - O$). This represented 2.75% ($|N - O|/|N|$) of the total number of non-lattice pairs in the 01/2010 version. On the other hand, 8,525 non-lattice pairs were found in the 07/2009 version but not 01/2010 ($O - N$), which amounted to 1.52% of the non-lattice pairs in the 07/2009 version. As can be seen from Fig. 4.11, the largest percentage change took place in the 03/2014 version (a total of 41,103 non-lattice pairs were added).

4.2.3 Potential Extensions

For large and complex ontological systems, exhaustive structural analysis tends to be time-consuming. For example, due to computational complexity, Jiang and Chute performed FCA-based analysis on only 10% of the possible candidates. Zhang and Bodenreider's lattice-based auditing method took almost three months to complete for a single version of SNOMED CT. It goes without saying that one would like to complete the automatic analysis as quickly as possible, so that the analytical results can be reviewed and validated in subsequent ontology auditing and quality assurance work.

Reimplementing Existing OQA Methods in the MapReduce Framework
We believe that semi-automatic and automated systematic methods reviewed in [28] for structural auditing could be considered to be reimplemented using the MapReduce framework. The benefits would be speed enhancement and scalability, so that we can afford time to analyze each version of the ontological system using the OQA method and compare conformance to the ontological principles, rules, and patterns underlying each method, over time. Section 4.2.1 can be seen as an exemplar to illustrate how this approach may work by implementing the lattice-based auditing method discussed in Sect. 4.1 using a MapReduce framework. In a similar way, Jiang and Chute's FCA-based method [76] for auditing the semantic completeness of SNOMED CT may be implemented using MapReduce so that exhaustive analysis can be obtained, rather than randomly selecting only 10% of the sample. One can imagine mapper and reducer jobs to construct massive amounts of local formal contexts in parallel, with FCA-tool ConExp again running in batch mode in parallel to achieve such an exhaustive analysis. Additionally, automated techniques to partition SNOMED CT into smaller groups of concepts using the area taxonomy and p-area taxonomy [88] could be scaled up using MapReduce to exhaustively pre-compute interesting taxonomy candidates for inspection. Basic ontological principles [26] can be systematically inspected for potential violation not only for individual ontological versions but for the entire collection of versions systematically over time. A by-product of this approach is that the aggregated "error-rate" against available ontological principles can be used as a quality measure, which hopefully improves over time.

Applying MaPLE-Like Approach to Other Ontologies

Our approach illustrated in Sect. 4.2.1, particularly MaPLE, has a few basic building blocks that are generally applicable.

One is to compute the transitive closure of a relation, in an unlabeled way (ignoring its specific relational types such as *is-a* or *part-of*), using MapReduce. This will ensure that the transitive property will never need to be recomputed in all subsequent steps, avoiding redundant processing and hence saving computational time.

The second is local closure, in the form of upper closure $(c, \uparrow c)$ or down closure $(c, \downarrow c)$. With transitive closure already pre-computed, obtaining upper closure and down closure is straightforward in MapReduce and can be efficiently implemented. If the reverse of a relation is needed, one can simply switch all pairs (x, y) to (y, x) to use, without having to pre-compute the reversed relationship.

Coupled with small-scale set operations, the upper closure and down closure can be used to compute the ontological fragment generated from any set of concept nodes X: the formula $\bigcup_{x,y \in X} (\uparrow x \cap \downarrow y)$ is first used to determine all the concept nodes in-between any two nodes x, y in X. Then, the relationships between the generated concept nodes are added by looking up the original ontological structure as input.

To perform evolutional change analysis on distinct versions of the same ontology, whether it is for basic changes such as the insertion and deletion of concepts and relationships, or for the changes in the result obtained by specific OQA methods, large-scale set-operations may be needed because of the size of the sets compared. This should be simple to address because there exist straightforward MapReduce algorithms for performing set operations such as intersection, union, and difference.

MaPLE-like analysis for extracting non-lattice pairs, reversals, and evolutional analysis, can be adapted for analyzing other ontological systems such as GO, FMA, or GALAN [89].

Conclusion: In this section, we presented our recent progresses made in using scalable cloud computing environment, Hadoop and MapReduce, to perform ontology quality assurance (OQA), and pointed to areas of future opportunity. Our contributions include: a general MapReduce lattice-checking algorithm for posets; an application of MaPLE for exhaustive analysis of SNOMED CT; and a global change analysis of SNOMED CT versions. Our approach sets the foundation for structural auditing of ontologies in a couple of new directions. One is to mine the large collection of non-lattice fragments to extract clinically interpretable insights in ontological evolution. The second is to perform large-scale MapReduce analysis of biomedical ontologies taking advantage of the combination of linguistic and structural information conveyed by the ontological systems, along the lines of work reported in Sect. 4.2.1.

To summarize, we would like to refer to "Big Data" as a frame of mind, or a "bigger vision," in perceiving the scientific landscape from a grander data scale, emboldened by the scalability of cloud computing, such as MapReduce, for massive parallel processing.

We demonstrated that such an approach can dramatically accelerate the speed of OQA analysis in cases of complex tasks that are less computationally feasible. We believe that such a scalable approach is beneficial for ontology quality assurance work in general, even for computationally feasible problems because it allows us to ask bigger questions and to answer them faster, putting computational barriers on the back of our minds so we can focus more on the scientific content.

4.3 Fast Non-lattice Detection and Algorithmic Correctness

This section introduces ANT-LCA, an algorithm for computing all non-trivial lowest common ancestors (LCA) of each pair of concepts in the graph induced by an ontological system. Here, the lowest common ancestors in the context of a graph are exactly the maximal shared descendants in the context of an ontology. In the remainder of the section, we discuss algorithms in graph-theoretic and order-theoretic terms. But whenever working with specific ontological examples, we switch back to maximal shared descendants. Distinct from existing approaches, ANT-LCA only computes LCAs for non-trivial pairs, those having at least one common ancestor. To skip all trivial pairs that may be of no practical interest, ANT-LCA employs a simple but innovative algorithmic strategy combining topological order and dynamic programming [47] to keep track of non-trivial pairs.

We provide correctness proofs and demonstrate about 2-orders of magnitude reduction, compared with the best parallel algorithms known to date, in computational time for two of the largest biomedical ontologies: SNOMED CT and Gene Ontology (GO). ANT-LCA achieved an average computation time of 30 and 3 seconds per version for SNOMED CT and GO, respectively, confirming our complexity analysis with a time-bound involving *pairability-degree* (i.e., the constant in big-O analysis of time-complexity) as a quadratic factor. ANT-LCA overcomes a fundamental computational barrier in subgraph analysis of ontological structures. It enables the implementation of a new breed of structural auditing methods that can not only identify potential problematic areas, but also automatically suggests specific changes that are needed to fix the quality issues.

4.3.1 LCA on Directed Acyclic Graphs

In a directed acyclic graph (DAG), a common ancestor (CA) of a pair of nodes u, v is a node w that is a shared ancestor of u, v. A lowest CA is a node w such that no other shared ancestor is closer (nearer) to u, v than w. A pair of nodes u, v is trivial if they do not have a shared ancestor, or one of them is the ancestor of the other. Conversely, non-trivial pairs are those having at least one lowest common ancestor other than the nodes already in the pair. Given a subset of nodes X in a DAG, we denote the set of lowest common ancestors of X

as $\mathsf{lca}(X)$, and common ancestors of X as $\mathsf{ca}(X)$, respectively. When X is a two-element set $\{a, b\}$ with two or more lowest common ancestors, it is called a *non-lattice pair.*

A pair of nodes (x, y) is called *pairable* if $\mathsf{lca}\{x, y\} \neq \emptyset$, $\mathsf{lca}\{x, y\} \neq \{x\}$, as well as $\mathsf{lca}\{x, y\} \neq \{y\}$. Intuitively, x, y is pairable if they share at least one non-trivial common ancestor. In this case, we also say that x is *pairable with* y, and (x, y) a *non-trivial* pair. We use notation $x \downarrow y$ to indicate that x is pairable with y. A *trivial pair* is a pair (x, y) that is not pairable. In fact, (x, y) is trivial if and only if $\mathsf{lca}\{x, y\} \subseteq \{x, y\}$, i.e., $\mathsf{lca}\{x, y\} = \emptyset$, $\mathsf{lca}\{x, y\} = \{x\}$, or $\mathsf{lca}\{x, y\} = \{y\}$. We write $\pi(u) = \{v \mid u \downarrow v\}$ for the set of all nodes v that are pairable with u.

4.3.2   The Computational Challenge

Exhaustive generation of non-lattice fragments for large ontological graphs such as SNOMED CT, with over 300,000 concepts and 450,000 *is-a* relations, is computationally expensive if not prohibitive, using an exhaustive sequential approach. For instance, in the approach discussed in Sect. 4.1, we employed SPARQL queries over an RDF representation of SNOMED CT, which took 3 months using standard desktop machines. In Sect. 4.2, we discuss a MapReduce pipeline for detecting non-lattice pairs for SNOMED CT, which took about 3 hours to complete using a Cloudera Hadoop cluster.

Our ANT-LCA algorithm provides a dramatic further reduction in computational time using sequential computation by using a strategy that *skips trivial pairs altogether, without even checking them.*

4.3.3   The ANT-LCA Algorithm

We present ANT-LCA in three components: initialization, pairability computation, and finding of shared ancestors embedded into pairability computation. We treat pairability computation separately to highlight ANT-LCA's core algorithmic insight without dealing with irrelevant overhead.

Initialization The initialization phase for ANT-LCA takes a DAG (V, E) as input and uses a modified version of topological sort [47] to obtain a topological order (index) for each node in V. This step takes linear time in $|V|$.

After initialization, we have two order relations on V: $\sqsubseteq$ and $\leq$. Here $\sqsubseteq$ (and the strict version $\sqsubset$) stands for the partial order determined by the input DAG (V, E) [47] (i.e., $v_1 \sqsubset v_2$ means there is an edge from v_1 to v_2). $\leq$ represents the usual arithmetic order on the topological index. By the property of topological sort, we have $u \sqsubset v$ implies $u < v$ for any $u, v \in V$.

Computing Pairability The core algorithmic idea of ANT-LCA is captured by the computation of the pairable function $p_i(u)$, intended to compute the function $\pi(u)$, where $p_i(u)$ is the set of nodes pairable with u computed up to step i, and $\pi(u)$ is the set of all nodes pairable with u. Algorithm 7 initializes $p_i(u)$ by fixing proper values for $p_0(u)$ for each $u \in V$. Algorithm 8 updates $p_i(u)$ as i gets incremented, in order to capture all nodes pairable with u at the completion of the algorithm.

Algorithm 7: Initialization phase for generating pairable sets. Here (V, E) is the input graph with V the set of nodes, and E the set of edges. $p_0(u)$ is the set of nodes pairable with u computed up to step 0 – the initialization step.

Input: (V, E) in topological order.
Output: Initialization of pairable elements
              for each node.

1 **for** $i \in V$ **do**
2   **for** $u \in i.to$ **do**
3 | $p_0(u) += i.to - \{u\}$;
4   **end**
5 **end**

In Algorithm 7, $i.to$ consists of all t such that $(i, t) \in E$. For each i, Algorithm 7 updates each u such that $(i, u) \in E$ by appending distinct members in $i.to$, such as v (Fig. 4.12, left) that are not comparable with u, into $p_0(u)$. Strictly speaking, for Algorithm 7 to be correct for arbitrary graphs, line 3 should be modified as $p_0(u) := i.to - \{x \mid u \sqsubseteq x\}$. This is, however, not necessary if nodes in $i.to$ are not comparable with each other, as is the case when the input graph has no "redundant" edges (when the *is-a* relation in an ontology is minimally represented without edges that are derivable from transitive closure).

Figure 4.12 (right) contains the Hasse diagram of an example DAG in topological order. The initialization results for $p_0(u)$ obtained by Algorithm 7 are displayed beside each node.

Algorithm 8 updates each i's upper neighbor u (lines 1 and 2) by adding those nodes that are pairable with i but not comparable with u (line 3). All nodes v that are pairable with i also gets updated by adjoining the upper neighbors of i to its set of pairable nodes (line 5). For abbreviation, the notation of relative set union ($\cup_x$) is used in Algorithm 8. For subsets A, B of V and $x \in V$, we write $A \cup_x B$ for $A \cup B$ while making sure that nodes in the resulting set are not comparable to x, i.e.,

$$A \cup_x B := (A - \{a \in A \mid x \sqsubseteq a \text{ or } a \sqsubseteq x\}) \cup (B - \{b \in B \mid x \sqsubseteq b \text{ or } b \sqsubseteq x\}).$$

In practice, one can take advantage of fast computation of transitive closure [90] and efficient disjoint union [91] for computing $A \cup_x B$.

Computing Common Ancestors of Non-trivial Pairs Algorithm 9 combines the computation of pairable nodes with the computation of (a subset of) their common ancestors $q_i(u, v)$, which contains their lowest common ancestors. The main ingredients of Algo-

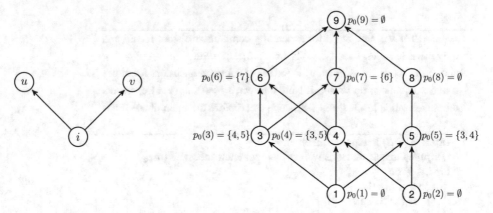

Fig. 4.12 Left: the iterative pattern for each edge $(i, u) \in E$. Right: initializing the pairable function for a graph consisting of topologically ordered nodes 1 to 9

rithm 9 is the addition of steps in lines 5, 13, and 14 which iteratively update common ancestors for pairable nodes (see Sect. 18 for the intermediate results of step-by-step run of Algorithm 9 on the example in Fig. 4.12). Note that Algorithm 9 does not guarantee that all common ancestors of u, v will eventually be included in $q_i(u, v)$, but it does include all lowest common ancestors of u, v (see Theorem 4.12 in Sect. 18). Therefore, an additional straightforward step is needed to extract the lowest elements in $q_i(u, v)$ to obtain $\mathsf{lca}\{u, v\}$.

Algorithm 8: Main steps for generating pairable sets. Here (V, E) is the input graph with V the set of nodes, and E the set of edges. $p_i(u)$ is the set of nodes pairable with u computed up to step i (> 0).

Input: (V, E) in topological order.
Output: The set of pairable nodes for each node.

1 **for** $i \in V$ **do**
2   **for** $u \in i.to$ **do**
3          $p_i(u) := p_{i-1}(u) \cup_u p_{i-1}(i)$
4   **end**
5   **for** $v \in p_{i-1}(i)$ **do**
6          $p_i(v) := p_{i-1}(v) \cup_v (i.to)$
7   **end**
8 **end**

Algorithm 9: Main steps for generating common ancestors for all and only pairable nodes. Here (V, E) is the input graph with V the set of nodes, and E the set of edges. $q_i(u, v)$ is the set of common ancestors for nodes u and v computed up to step i. Note that when $i = 0$, $q_0(u, v)$ represents the initialization result (lines 1-8), computed before the main phase (lines 9-18).

Input: (V, E) in topological order.
Output: Pairable nodes as well as their common ancestors (in q_i).

1 **for** $i \in V$ **do**
2   **for** $u \in i.to$ **do**
3        $p_0(u) := i.to - \{u\}$
4   **for** $v \in i.to$ with $u \neq v$ **do**
5           $q_0(u, v) := q_0(u, v) \cup \{i\};$
6   **end**
7   **end**
8 **end**
9 **for** $i \in V$ **do**
10   **for** $u \in i.to$ **do**
11       $p_i(u) := p_{i-1}(u) \cup_u p_{i-1}(i)$
12   **for** $v \in p_{i-1}(i)$ **do**
13          $q_i(u, v) := q_{i-1}(u, v) \cup q_{i-1}(i, v);$
14          $q_i(v, u) := q_i(u, v);$
15          $p_i(v) := p_{i-1}(v) \cup_v (i.to)$
16   **end**
17   **end**
18 **end**

Illustrative Example Although using only a small number of steps, the recursive nature involved in Algorithm 9 as well as the intricate behavior can be better demonstrated through an example. The following figures illustrate a step-by-step run of Algorithm 9 on the example in Fig. 4.12. Edges being iterated and incremental value changes are highlighted in blue.

Updating up to node 3 and edge $(3, 6)$ gives the result illustrated in Fig. 4.13. Note that nothing gets updated when $i = 1, 2$. When $i = 3$, $u = 6$, $v = 4$, since nodes 6 and 4 are not pairable, nothing gets updated. When $i = 3$, $u = 6$, $v = 5$, since nodes 6 and 5 are pairable, we have $p_3(6) = \{5, 7\}$, $p_3(5) = \{3, 4, 6\}$, $q_3(6, 5) = q_3(5, 6) = \{1\}$.

As shown in Fig. 4.14, for $i = 3$, $u = 7$, $v = 4$, since nodes 7 and 4 are not pairable, no updates took place. For $i = 3$, $u = 7$, $v = 5$, since $p_3(7) = \{5, 6\}$ and $p_3(5) = \{3, 4, 6, 7\}$, we have $q_3(7, 5) = q_3(5, 7) = \{1\}$.

Figure 4.15 captures the snapshot for $i = 4$ and $u = 6$: when $v = 3$, we have nodes 6 and 3 are not pairable and no update is needed; when $v = 5$, we have $q_4(6, 5) = q_4(5, 6) = \{1, 2\}$.

Figure 4.16 shows the step for $i = 4$ and $u = 7$: when $v = 3$, we have nodes 7 and 3 are not pairable; when $v = 5$, the updated result is $q_4(5, 7) = q_4(7, 5) = \{1, 2\}$.

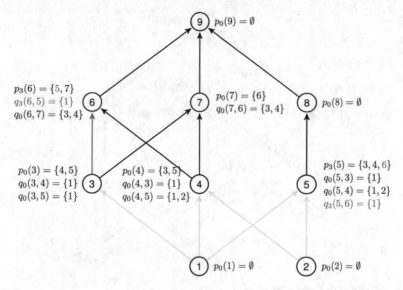

Fig. 4.13 Updating up to node 3 and edge (3, 6)

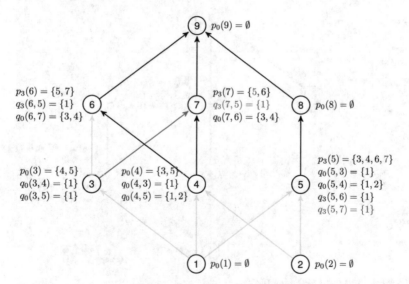

Fig. 4.14 Step for node 3 and edge (3, 7)

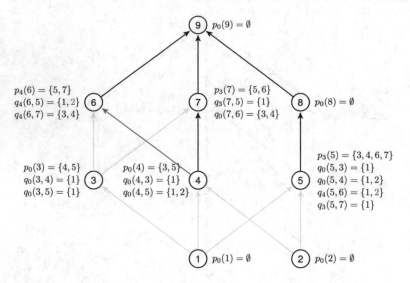

Fig. 4.15 Step for node 4 and edge (4, 6)

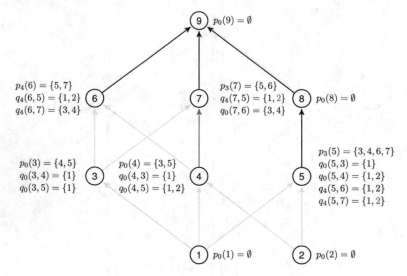

Fig. 4.16 Step for node 4 and edge (4, 7)

Figure 4.17 captures the following configurations. $i = 5, u = 8, v = 3$: $p_5(3) = \{4, 5, 8\}$, $p_5(8) = \{3\}$, $q_5(3, 8) = q_5(8, 3) = \{1\}$; $i = 5, u = 8, v = 4$: $p_5(4) = \{3, 5, 8\}$, $p_5(8) = \{3, 4\}$, $q_5(8, 4) = q_5(4, 8) = \{1, 2\}$; $i = 5, u = 8, v = 6$: $p_5(8) = \{3, 4, 6\}$, $p_5(6) = \{5, 7, 8\}$, $q_5(8, 6) = q_5(6, 8) = \{1, 2\}$; $i = 5, u = 8, v = 7$: $p_5(8) = \{3, 4, 6, 7\}$, $p_5(7) = \{5, 6, 8\}$, $q_5(8, 7) = q_5(7, 8) = \{1, 2\}$.

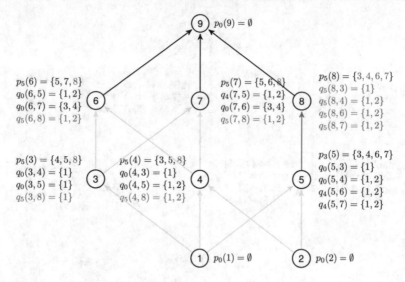

Fig. 4.17 Step for node 5 and edge (5, 8)

Finally, Fig. 4.18 shows that for $i = 6, 7, 8$, nothing gets updated since node 9 is not pairable to any other node.

Correctness of the Algorithm

We establish the correctness of Algorithms 8 and 17 in a sequence of lemmas and theorems.

With respect to a topologically sorted input graph (V, E), we distinguish the set $\pi(u)$ of all nodes pairable with u, and $p_i(u)$, the dynamic store of nodes pairable with u *at a stage i of the algorithm*. In the remainder of the section we refer to nodes in V solely by their topological indices, integers that can also be incremented for algorithmic iteration in a while-loop.

According to Algorithm 8, $p_i(u)$ has the following straightforward properties:

- Monotonicity: for all $w \in V$, for all $i \le j \in V$, we have $p_i(w) \subseteq p_j(w)$;
- Symmetry: for all $u, v \in V$, for all $i \in V$, $u \in p_i(v)$ implies $v \in p_i(u)$;
- Diagonality: for all $v \in V$, $p_v(v) = p_{v-1}(v)$.

Since Algorithm 8 initializes and grows $p_i(u)$ with only nodes pairable with u, we have

Theorem 4.3 *For all $u \in V$, for all $i \in V$,*

$$p_i(u) \subseteq \pi(u).$$

For proving containment in the other direction the next three lemmas serve as building blocks. Notationally, we use $[x, y]$ to stand for the closed integer interval $\{i \mid x \le i \le y\}$.

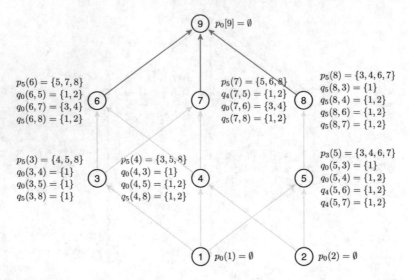

Fig. 4.18 For node $i = 6, 7, 8$, nothing gets updated since node 9 is not pairable to any other node

Lemma 4.4 *Suppose* $b \in \mathrm{lca}(u, v)$ *and* $(b, u) \in E$. *For* $i \in [0, n]$, *let* $(v_i, v_{i+1}) \in E$ *be edges such that* $b = v_0$ *and* $v_n = v$. *Then* $u \in p_{v_{(i-1)}}(v_i)$ *for all* $i \in [1, n]$.

Lemma 4.5 *Let* $(v_i, v_{i+1}) \in E$ *be edges in* (V, E) *for* $i \in [0, n]$, *with* $b = v_0$ *and* $v_n = v$. *Suppose* $\mathrm{lca}(x, v) = b$ *and* $x \in \pi(v_i)$ *for* $i \in [0, n]$. *If* $x \in p_{v_k}(v_{k+1})$ *for some* k, *then* $x \in p_{v_j}(v_{j+1})$ *for all* $j \in [k, n]$.

Lemma 4.6 *For all* $0 < i < n$, *we have* $p_{v_i}(v_i) \subseteq p_{v_i}(v_{i+1})$, *and moreover* $p_{v_i}(v_i) \subseteq p_{v_{(i+1)}}(v_{i+1})$, *by monotonicity*.

Lemmas 4.4, 4.5, and 4.6 show how pairability information is propagated along a path. Next we deal with the general situation of how this information is propagated to a pair of (pairable) nodes starting from the initial setting. To do so, consider a subgraph $D = A \cup B$ of (V, E), with $A = \{u_i \mid i \in [1, m]\}$ and $B = \{v_j \mid j \in [1, n]\}$ such that (u_{i-1}, u_i) and (v_{j-1}, v_j) are distinct edges with $i \in [1, m]$ and $j \in [1, n]$, where (see Fig. 4.19)

1. $u_0 = v_0$, $u_m = u$, and $v_n = v$,
2. $u \in \pi(v)$ and $u_0 \in \mathrm{lca}(u, v)$, and
3. $A \cap B = \emptyset$.

Consider $W = \{w_i \mid i \in [1, m + n]\} = A \cup B$, with topological indices appearing in $A \cup B$ sorted in ascending order.

Fig. 4.19 Subgraph with $A = \{u_i \mid i \in [1, m]\}$ and $B = \{v_j \mid j \in [1, n]\}$

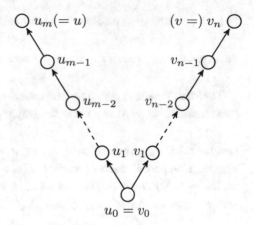

Definition 4.7 The i-th alternation index for W is the index α_i, such that either $w_{\alpha_i} \in A$ but $w_{\alpha_i+1} \in B$, or $w_{\alpha_i} \in B$ but $w_{\alpha_i+1} \in A$.

The next lemma characterizes how pairability information "jumps" from one branch (say A) to the other (say B) at critical junctures of an alternation index.

Lemma 4.8 *For any alternation index α_i, we have: 1. if $v_t = w_{\alpha_i}$ and $u_s = w_{\alpha_i+1}$ then $u_s \in p_{v_t}(v_t)$; 2. if $u_s = w_{\alpha_i}$ and $v_t = w_{\alpha_i+1}$ then $v_t \in p_{u_s}(u_s)$.*

The following Theorem 4.9 deals with the opposite direction of Theorem 4.3. It allows us to conclude that for each $u \in V$, if $v \in \pi(u)$ then there exists $i \in V$, such that $v \in p_i(u)$ by choosing a large enough i. With it, all nodes pairable with u are accounted for by the function $p_i(u)$.

Theorem 4.9 *For all $i \in V$ and for all $w \leq i$, we have*

$$p_i(w) \supseteq \pi(w) \cap [1, i],$$

where $[1, i]$ stands for the integer interval $\{j \mid 1 \leq j \leq i\}$.

Similar to $p_i(u)$, the binary function $q_i(u, v)$ has the following properties, as can be directly derived from Algorithm 9:

- Monotonicity: for all $u, v \in V$, for all $i \leq j \in V$, we have $q_i(u, v) \subseteq q_j(u, v)$;
- Symmetry: for all $u, v \in V$, for all $i \in V$, we have $q_i(u, v) = q_i(v, u)$;
- Diagonality: For all $u, v \in V$, we have $q_u(u, v) = q_{u-1}(u, v)$.

By inspecting steps involved in Algorithm 9, we can establish this fact:

Theorem 4.10 *For each $i \in V$ and for each $u \in \pi(v)$, we have $q_i(u, v) \subseteq \mathsf{ca}\{u, v\}$.*

The next lemma shows how alternation indices help propagate the common ancestor information to all relevant pairs in the graph.

Lemma 4.11 *Suppose $x \in \mathsf{lca}\{u, v\}$, $u \in \pi(v)$, and suppose that (see Fig. 4.19) (u_{i-1}, u_i) and (v_{j-1}, v_j) are distinct edges with $i \in [1, m]$ and $j \in [1, n]$, where $x = u_0 = v_0$, $u_m = u$, and $v_n = v$. For any alternation index α_i as given in Definition 4.7, we have 1. if $w_{\alpha_i} = v_t$ and $w_{\alpha_i+1} = u_s$, then $x \in q_{v_t}(v_t, u_s)$; 2. if $w_{\alpha_i} = u_t$ and $w_{\alpha_i+1} = v_s$, then $x \in q_{u_t}(u_t, v_s)$.*

Lemma 4.11 leads to the following theorem, which affirms the correctness of Algorithm 9.

Theorem 4.12 *Suppose $x \in \mathsf{lca}\{u, v\}$ with $u \in \pi(v)$. Then either $x \in q_u(u, v)$ or $x \in q_v(u, v)$.*

Theorem 4.12 shows that Algorithm 9 finds all lowest common ancestors of u, v in $q_i(u, v)$, for some i. It does not, however, guarantee that all common ancestors of u, v will eventually be included in $q_i(u, v)$. Neither does Algorithm 9 ensure that all elements in $q_i(u, v)$ are LCAs of u and v. Therefore, an additional straightforward step is needed to extract the lowest elements in $q_i(u, v)$ after the termination of Algorithm 9, to obtain $\mathsf{lca}\{u, v\}$.

4.3.4 Experiments on SNOMED CT and Gene Ontology

ANT-LCA was implemented in Java based on JDK7. Experiments on SNOMED CT and GO were performed on a MacBook Pro running Mac OS X Yosemite, with 16 GB RAM and Intel Core i7 processor. For a detailed discussion and analysis of results, please see [92].

SNOMED CT

We applied this approach to the 07/2012 version containing 296,433 concepts and 440,049 direct *is-a* relations connecting concepts. Among all possible concept pairs, 150,639 were identified as pairable after the initialization step in Algorithm 7, a total of 1,383,888 were detected as pairable, among which 578,237 were found to be non-lattice pairs. It took 28 seconds (averaged over 10 runs) to compute non-lattice pairs and 524 seconds (averaged over 5 runs) to compute non-lattice fragments.

Gene Ontology

We applied this approach to the 02/2016 version of the Gene Ontology containing a total of 44,222 concepts and 72,742 direct *is-a* relations connecting concepts. Among all possible concept pairs, 3,642 were identified as pairable after the initialization step in Algorithm 7, a total of 328,760 were detected as pairable, among which 102,948 were found to be non-lattice pairs. It took 3 seconds to compute non-lattice pairs and 32 seconds to compute non-lattice fragments.

4.3.5 Further Analysis of the Approach

Time Complexity for Algorithm 8

Let σ_G be the *pairability degree* of graph G, defined as $\max_{u \in V} \pi(u)$, i.e., the maximum number of pairable nodes a single node can have in graph G. Algorithm 8 involves a main iteration process over all edges $(i, u) \in E$ of the input graph, as given in lines 1 and 2. Then the time complexity for line 3 is (using set union complexity)

$$\sum_{(i,u)\in E} |p_i(u)|,$$

which is bounded by (with the assumption that the union cost is proportional to the size of the resulting set [91])

$$\sum_{(i,u)\in E} |\pi(u)|.$$

Hence,

$$\sum_{(i,u)\in E} |p_i(u)| \leq \sigma_G \cdot |E|.$$

Similarly, the time complexity for lines 4 and 5 is

$$\sum_{(i,u)\in E} \sum_{v \in p_{i-1}(i)} |p_i(v)|.$$

We have

$$\sum_{(i,u)\in E} \sum_{v \in p_{i-1}(i)} |p_i(v)| \leq \sigma_G^2 \cdot |E|.$$

Therefore, the overall time-complexity of Algorithm 8 is bounded by $\sigma_G^2 \cdot |E|$. Space complexity is similarly bounded, but less of a concern here due to the availability of sufficiently large, standard sizes of RAMs. For sparse graphs with small σ_G, Algorithm 8 performs well, as our experimental result in the next section shows. In the worst case, $\sigma_G = |V|$, and the running time in the worst case is $O(|V|^2 \cdot |E|)$ and is the same as brute force search. In the best case σ_G is a constant, and the running time in the base case is $O(|E|)$. The actual time needed for the algorithm, $\sum_{(i,u)\in E} \sum_{v \in p_{i-1}(i)} |p_i(v)|$, is very close to the best case for the data set in our experiments. Even though σ_G may be in the thousands, the average size of $\pi(v)$, a more realistic estimation for the actual computational time, is below 50.

Intuitively, the more tree-like the input ontology is, the closer to the best case time-complexity of $O(|E|)$ our algorithm will achieve. The worst cases are when every pair of nodes are pairable, achievable when the ontology is dense with shared descendant concepts among its concept nodes.

Time Complexity for Algorithm 9
Note that we intentionally nested the for-loop in lines 4–6 of Algorithm 8, to faithfully account for the time-complexity for Algorithm 9. For Algorithm 9, the double nesting is necessary in order to compute pairable pairs while accumulating common ancestors (between u and v). If we are interested only in computing pairability, then the nesting in lines 4–6 of Algorithm 8 is not necessary, and we obtain a better time-complexity of $\sigma_G \cdot (|E| + |V|)$.

The key steps involved in Algorithm 9 can be captured by Algorithm 8 except for the accumulation of common ancestors in steps 13 and 14. We assume the computation required for these two steps to be a constant by keeping up to two LCAs, in order to provide a fair comparison with existing algorithms (which only output a representative LCA for each pair). Therefore, the time-complexity of Algorithm 8 is also bounded by $\sigma_G^2 \cdot |E|$. Therefore, the best case and worst case analyses for Algorithm 8 apply to Algorithm 9 as well.

Related Work on LCA
Many attempts have been made to improve the efficiency of algorithms for the all-pairs all-LCA problem [93, 94], i.e., finding all LCAs associated with each pair of nodes. More recently, Dash et al. [95] presented an approach that combines the efficiency of existing LCA algorithms on trees with range-interval labeling scheme and an efficient matrix multiplication. This approach achieves near-linear time for tree-like, rooted DAGs, but query results are limited to a single representative LCA per each pair of nodes. This is a limit for applications that require all-LCAs as query results. In general, the all-pairs all-LCA problem remains to be super-quadratic, since its time-complexity is inherently tied to algorithms for matrix-multiplication [94, 96]. For many DAGs arising in real-world applications such SNOMED CT (with over 300,000 nodes), existing algorithms become impractical.

In general approaches to the LCA problem, one distinguishes the off-line and online computations. Off-line computation serves to preprocess the input graph in order to speedup online LCA queries. Our section focuses on off-line processing in order to support constant online query for a representative LCA, or online query for all LCAs (with performance parameterized in the size of the resulting set).

A key distinction of ANT-LCA from existing approaches is that it ensures computation is performed on all and only non-trivial pairs. In fact, the time complexity of ANT-LCA is determined by the number of non-trivial pairs in the input graph, as our complexity analysis shows. Using the average size of pairable pairs for a given node, which is a more realistic reflection of the actual computational time, the time complexity for our experimental cases is approximately $(50)^2 \cdot |E|$.

Another distinction of our approach is that we compute all LCAs (of all non-trivial pairs) instead of a representative LCA. This makes our task more computationally intensive, and also makes many existing approaches to the LCA problem inapplicable. Our all LCA requirement is motivated by real-world application needs for implementing lattice-based approach to ontology quality assurance. Compared with the fastest all pairs representative LCA algorithm known to date with an $O(|V| \cdot |E|)$ time complexity [95], ANT-LCA provides a rough speed-up of three orders of magnitude for SNOMED CT. However, the worst time-complexity for our algorithm, $|V|^2 \cdot |E|$, is attained when virtually all nodes are pairable with all other nodes.

Limitations

Since ANT-LCA is designed for detecting the lowest common ancestors for all non-trivial pairs in a DAG, it is generally applicable to other ontologies or terminologies which are hierarchically organized in a DAG. We have applied it to SNOMED CT, Gene Ontology, and NCI Thesaurus for ontology quality assurance.

There are two types of limitations. One is specific to the ANT-LCA algorithm, and the other is related to the non-lattice approach. The limitation of the ANT-LCA algorithm is that, although it is efficient and suitable for ontological graph structures that are tree-like, it may not work well with other types of graph structures when all pairs of nodes are pairable.

Limitations of the non-lattice approach include the following. (1): The approach may not be efficient for ontologies that are "shallow," such as Ontology for General Medical Science (maximum depth 6), BRENDA Tissue and Enzyme Source Ontology (maximum depth 6), and Current Procedural Terminology (maximum depth 7), from BioPortal. (2): Our algorithm itself is agnostic to relation types, so it will still work for such relations as *part-of*. However, the non-lattice approach is not applicable to other types of relations since this approach is only meaningful for the *is-a* hierarchy (of any ontology) due to its theoretical underpinning-based Formal Concept Analysis. We are not aware of any (theoretical) reasons that indicate non-lattice fragments to be problematic for other types of relations. However, this should not diminish the value of our non-lattice approach.

Conclusion: To summarize, this section introduced an efficient algorithm for detecting non-lattice pairs and generating non-lattice fragments for ontology quality assurance work. Our algorithm overcomes a fundamental computational barrier in sub-graph based structural analysis of large ontological systems. It enables the implementation of a new breed of structural auditing methods that not only identifies potential problematic areas, but also automatically suggests changes to fix the issues.

Non-lattice Substructures in Ontological Analysis 5

This chapter presents a variety of approaches that leverage non-lattice substructures (i.e. non-lattice fragments or non-lattice subgraphs) for ontological analyses.

5.1 Substructure Embedding Between Ontologies

A structural disparity of the subsumption relationship between FMA and SNOMED CT's *Body Structure* sub-hierarchy is that while the *is-a* relation in FMA has a tree structure, the corresponding relation in *Body Structure* is not even a lattice. This section introduces a method called NEO for the non-lattice embedding of FMA fragments into the *Body Structure* sub-hierarchy to understand (1) this structural disparity and (2) its potential utility in analyzing non-lattice fragments in SNOMED CT. NEO consists of four steps. First, transitive, upper- and down-closures are computed for FMA and SNOMED CT using MapReduce, a modern scalable distributed computing technique. Secondly, UMLS mappings between FMA and SNOMED CT concepts are used to identify equivalent concepts in non-lattice fragments from *Body Structure*. Then, non-lattice fragments in the *Body Structure* sub-hierarchy are extracted, and FMA concepts matching those in the non-lattice fragments are used as the seeds to generate the corresponding FMA fragments. Lastly, the corresponding FMA fragments are embedded to the non-lattice fragments for comparative visualization and analysis. After identifying 8,428 equivalent concepts between the collection of over 30,000 concepts in *Body Structure* and the collection of over 83,000 concepts in FMA using UMLS equivalent concept mappings, 2,117 shared *is-a* relations and 5,715 mismatched relations were found. Among *Body Structure*'s 90,465 non-lattice fragments, 65,968 (73%) contained one or more *is-a* relations that are in SNOMED CT but not in FMA, even though they have equivalent source and target concepts. This shows that SNOMED CT may be more liberal in classifying a relation as *is-a*, a potential explanation for the fragments not conforming to the lattice property.

© The Author(s), under exclusive license to Springer Nature Switzerland AG 2022   109
G.-Q. Zhang et al., *Formal Methods for the Analysis of Biomedical Ontologies*,
Synthesis Lectures on Data, Semantics, and Knowledge,
https://doi.org/10.1007/978-3-031-12131-9_5

Fig. 5.1 Example of matching
concepts in FMA and
SNOMED CT without
matching relations between
them. The numbers indicated
below the labels are identifiers
in the respective systems

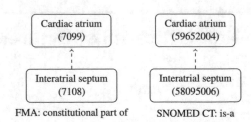

FMA: constitutional part of   SNOMED CT: is-a

SNOMED CT is the most comprehensive clinical terminology system used worldwide.
Foundational Model of Anatomy (FMA) provides a unifying framework for the nature of the
diverse entities for human anatomy. However, SNOMED CT and FMA are not in complete
agreement when it comes to the usage of *is-a* classification. For example (Fig. 5.1), both
the concepts "*Cardiac atrium*" and "*Interatrial septum*" are in SNOMED CT and in FMA,
as mapped by UMLS. While the relation "*Interatrial septum*" *is-a* "*Cardiac atrium*" is
asserted in SNOMED CT, FMA does not include this relation. Instead, FMA asserts a
different relation only: "*Interatrial septum*" is a *constitutional part of* "*Cardiac atrium*."

   The purpose of this section is to provide a systematic study of such a structural disparity
between FMA and SNOMED CT, motivated by the observation that the *is-a* relation in
FMA has a tree structure, but the corresponding relation in SNOMED CT is not even
a lattice. We introduce a method called NEO, Non-Lattice Embedding of Ontologies, for
systematic structural embedding of FMA fragments into the *Body Structure* sub-hierarchy, to
understand this structural disparity and its potential utility in analyzing non-lattice fragments
in SNOMED CT.

5.1.1   Steps for Non-lattice Embedding

Our method NEO for non-lattice embedding of ontologies consists of four steps. First, transitive, upper- and down-closures are computed for FMA v3.1 and SNOMED CT's *Body Structure* (03/2014 version) using MapReduce. Secondly, equivalent concepts between FMA and
SNOMED CT's *Body Structure* are identified using UMLS mappings. Thirdly, non-lattice
fragments in the *Body Structure* sub-hierarchy are extracted, and FMA concepts matching
non-lattice fragments are used as the seeds to generate the corresponding FMA fragments.
Lastly, the corresponding FMA fragments are embedded to the non-lattice fragments for
comparative visualization and analysis.

Computing Closures
Given a concept c in an ontology, we use $c^{\uparrow}$ and $c^{\downarrow}$ to denote its upper-closure and down-
closure respectively, with respect to the hierarchical order of the ontology. By "c's upper-
closure" we mean all the ancestors of c excluding itself, and by "c's down-closure" we mean
all the descendants of c, excluding itself. For SNOMED CT's *Body Structure*, the transitive,
upper- and down-closures are calculated in terms of the *is-a* relation. For FMA, the relations

including *part of*, *regional part of*, *constitutional part of*, *systemic part of*, *member of*, and *branch of* are also used to calculate the closures in addition to the *is-a* relation. These relations are included in order to provide a reference point for the relationships between matched concepts in non-lattice fragments and their corresponding FMA fragments. Such closures are also used directly for the rendering and analysis of embedded (or merged) fragments.

Sequential algorithms for computing transitive closures, such as Floyd-Warshall algorithm, has a cubic time complexity. Therefore, it is time-consuming to use it for large ontological structures such as SNOMED CT (>300 k concepts, >450 k *is-a* relations) and FMA (>83 k of concepts, >2.5 m of relations). We develop a parallel, distributed algorithm to compute transitive closure using MapReduce. This algorithm consists of two main steps. First, a hash map of concepts and their direct parents are stored in each computing node. Then in the map phase, each mapper reads in a concept and recursively collects its ancestors, level by level, until no direct parents can be found. In the reduce phase, each reducer emits all concept-ancestor pairs. Computing transitive closure for *Body Structure* and FMA each took less than 30 seconds. Also, upper- and down-closures are calculated using MapReduce to generate concept-closure pairs $(c, c^\uparrow)$ and $(c, c^\downarrow)$, which are used for generating a fragment from any given collection of seed concepts.

Identifying Equivalent Concepts Using UMLS
We use the distribution file *MRCONSO* provided by UMLS (2014AA release) to extract equivalent concepts between SNOMED CT and FMA. A concept in SNOMED CT and a concept in FMA are considered equivalent if they share the same CUI. A total of 8,428 equivalent concepts are identified. These equivalent concepts are used to extract FMA fragments corresponding to the non-lattice fragments in SNOMED CT's *Body Structure*, as described in the following subsection.

Extracting Non-lattice Fragments for SNOMED CT's Body Structure Sub-hierarchy
We use non-lattice pairs and their maximal lower bounds identified for SNOMED CT's *Body Structure* in Sect. 4.2 to generate non-lattice fragments. Given a non-lattice concept pair $C = \{c_1, c_2\}$ and the set L of their maximal lower bounds, the corresponding non-lattice fragment is computed using the formula:

$$C \cup L \cup \bigcup_{c \in C, l \in L} \{c^\downarrow \cap l^\uparrow\} \tag{5.1}$$

Since there are 90,465 non-lattice pairs, a sequential approach to computing non-lattice fragments may take several hours. To speed up, we generate non-lattice fragments in parallel using MapReduce:

- First, two hash maps are distributed to every computing node. One hash map stores concepts and their upper-closures, and the other hash map stores concepts and their down-closures.

- Then, in the map phase, each mapper reads in a non-lattice concept pair C and their maximal lower bounds L, finds down-closures for the concepts in C and upper-closures for the concepts in L from the hash maps and performs set operations to obtain the non-lattice fragment.
- Finally, in the reduce phase, each reducer emits the non-lattice pairs and their non-lattice fragments.

Extracting Corresponding FMA Fragments After equivalent concepts in FMA and SNOMED CT's *Body Structure* sub-hierarchy are identified, we find all matching concepts in FMA for each non-lattice fragment in *Body Structure*. Using these matching concepts as seeds, we construct the corresponding FMA fragment in the following way. Suppose S is the set of FMA concepts matched with those in a non-lattice fragment. First, we identify the maximal and minimal of concepts in S by the formulas $S - \bigcup_{s \in S} s^{\downarrow}$ and $S - \bigcup_{s \in S} s^{\uparrow}$, respectively. Then the corresponding FMA fragment is obtained similarly to Eq. (5.1) for computing a non-lattice fragment.

Embedding FMA Fragments to Non-lattice Fragments

Given a non-lattice fragment in SNOMED CT's *Body Structure*, the corresponding FMA fragment is embedded to the non-lattice fragment to visualize and compare the structures of the two fragments. For the embedding (or merging) of the two fragments, we not only need the matched concepts from both fragments, but also the matching relations. When mapping the relations, we distinguish matched *is-a* and mismatched *is-a* relation. A matched *is-a* relation is one that is in both SNOMED CT and FMA. A mismatched *is-a* relation is one that is in SNOMED CT but not in FMA (which could be relations other than *is-a*). Then, we merge the two fragments (both concepts and relations) together and render them using topological sort, a well-known rendering algorithm for directed acyclic graphs. The rendering of the merged fragments is implemented using the svg (scalable vector graphics) drawing library D3 (http://www.d3js.org) (see Fig. 5.3 for an example of the merged fragments).

5.1.2   Results Obtained and Visualization

Matched Concepts and Relations

A total of 8,428 equivalent concepts were identified among over 30,000 concepts in SNOMED CT's *Body Structure* and over 83,000 concepts in FMA. To illustrate, in Fig. 5.2, concepts 1, 3, 5, 7 in SNOMED CT are equivalent to concepts 2, 4, 6, 8 in FMA, respectively. We also identified 7,832 relations having equivalent source and target concepts between SNOMED CT's *Body Structure* and FMA. Among these 7,832 relations, 2,117 (27%) are *is-a* relations in both SNOMED CT and FMA (i.e., matched), and 5,715 are *is-a* relations in SNOMED CT but not *is-a* relations in FMA (i.e., mismatched). As illustrated in Fig. 5.2, the *is-a* relation between concepts 1 and 3 in SNOMED CT is matched with the *is-a* relation

Fig. 5.2 Summary of matching/mismatching results

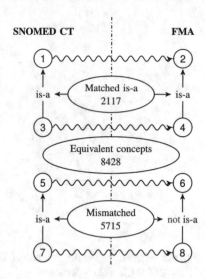

between 2 and 4 in FMA, but the *is-a* relation between concepts 5 and 7 in SNOMED CT is mismatched with non *is-a* relation between 6 and 8 in FMA.

Mismatched Relations in Non-lattice Fragments

Among 90,465 non-lattice fragments in SNOMD CT's *Body Structure* identified in Sect. 4.2, 65,968 (73%) contained one or more *is-a* relations that are in SNOMED CT but not in FMA, even though they have equivalent source and target concepts. This shows that SNOMED CT may be more liberal in classifying a relation as subsumption, which may cause the fragments not conforming the lattice property. Figure 5.4 shows 10 frequently mismatched relations in SNOMED CT (*is-a*) and FMA (not *is-a*). For example, the relationship of "*Structure of pelvic viscus*" and "*Structure of abdominal viscus*" has a *is-a* relation in SNOMED CT, but *member of* relation in FMA.

Visualization of Merged Fragments

Figure 5.3 displays the merged ontological fragments determined by the non-lattice pair "*Cardiac chamber*" (91744000) and "*Cardiac septum*" (10746000) in SNOMED CT's *Body Structure*. The blue nodes and edges represent concepts and *is-a* relations in SNOMED CT, respectively. The red nodes and edges represent concepts and *is-a* relations in FMA, the green edges represent other relations in FMA. The gray nodes and edges represent matched concepts and *is-a* relations between SNOMED CT and FMA. The dotted gray edges represent non-exact matching relations between them, that is, *is-a* relations in SNOMED CT but other relations in FMA. There is no blue node in Fig. 5.3, since all the concepts in the non-lattice fragment determined by the given non-lattice pair have matched concepts in FMA.

It can be seen from Fig. 5.3 that the pair "*Cardiac chamber*" and "*Cardiac septum*" has three maximal common descendants: "*Interventricular septum,*" "*Atrioventricular septum,*"

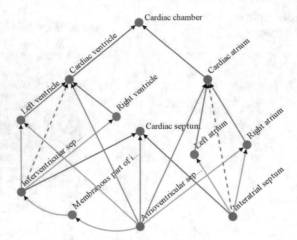

Fig. 5.3 Merged graph after embedding the corresponding FMA fragment to a non-lattice fragment in SNOMED CT's *Body Structure*

1. Structure of pelvic viscus (8279000) *member of* Structure of abdominal viscus (19203006)
2. Small intestinal structure (30315005) *regional part of* Intestinal structure (113276009)
3. Uterine structure (35039007) *member of* Structure of pelvic viscus (8279000)
4. Penile structure (18911002) *regional part of* Male external genitalia structure (90418005)
5. Chest wall structure (78904004) *constitutional part of* Thoracic structure (51185008)
6. Male internal genitalia structure (38242008) *regional part of* Male genital structure (90264002)
7. Large intestinal structure (14742008) *regional part of* Intestinal structure (113276009)
8. Pelvic wall structure (3665003) *constitutional part of* Pelvic structure (12921003)
9. Abdominal wall structure (83908009) *constitutional part of* Abdominal structure (113345001)
10. Endometrial structure (2739003) *constitutional part of* Structure of uterine wall (245485002)

Fig. 5.4 10 frequently mismatched relations in FMA occurring in non-lattice fragments in SNOMED CT as *is-a* relation

and "*Interatrial septum*." It is worth noting that removing any of the dotted gray edges or blue edges will reduce the number of maximal lower bounds. For example, removing the dotted *is-a* relation from "*Interatrial septum*" to "*Cardiac septum*" will result in two (instead of three) maximal common descendants in SNOMED CT. If mismatched *is-a* relations are removed in Fig. 5.3, we obtain a lattice conforming fragment.

For further details, please see [97].

Conclusion: This section presented NEO, a systematic method to structurally embed FMA fragments into SNOMED CT's *Body Structure* sub-hierarchy using non-lattice fragments. 73% of non-lattice fragments contain *is-a* relations that are not found in FMA. This shows that SNOMED CT is more liberal in classifying a relation as subsumption, a potential reason for inducing non-lattice fragments in *Body Structure*.

5.2   Concept Labels in Non-lattice Fragments

In this section, we introduce a novel approach to systematically identifying inconsistencies, such as missing hierarchical relations and concepts in SNOMED CT and NCIt, based on the structural properties of non-lattice subgraphs and the lexical properties of concept labels involved in these subgraphs. We extend our earlier work on non-lattice subgraphs by incorporating lexical patterns to precisely identify error types, along with suggestions for remediation. Compared to other methods developed for quality assurance in both the ontologies, the main difference in this approach is that other methods only identify potential errors, while we also provide remediation for the errors identified.

5.2.1   Steps to Identify Potential Errors and Propose Remediations

Our approach to identifying potential errors in SNOMED CT and NCIt can be summarized as follows. We identify non-lattice pairs in both the ontologies and generate the corresponding non-lattice subgraphs. We identify lexical patterns indicative of missing concepts or hierarchical relations, which we apply to the non-lattice subgraphs. Finally, experts evaluate a sample of the potential errors detected, as well as the proposed remediation. We used the distribution files of the September 2015 version of SNOMED CT (U.S. edition) and 16.12d version of NCIt.

Identifying Lexical Patterns Indicative of Missing Concepts and Relations
Because it is impractical to manually review large numbers of non-lattice subgraphs, we introduce an automatic approach leveraging additional lexical information (concept names) to identify lexical patterns in non-lattice subgraphs indicative of certain types of errors. We consider the fully specified name of a SNOMED CT concept and the preferred term of a NCIt concept c as a set (bag) of words in lower-case c. For instance, the fully specified name of the SNOMED CT concept ID *235838003*, (c), is "*Irritable bowel syndrome variant of childhood*," and its set of words, $\{c\}$, is *irritable, bowel, syndrome, variant, of, childhood*. Utilizing the information of sets of words for concepts in the upper and lower bounds, we define four patterns indicative of a situation where hierarchical relations or intermediary concepts may be missing.

Containment The set of words for one concept in the upper bounds is contained in the set of words for another concept in the upper bounds; or the set of words for one concept in the lower bounds is contained in the set of words for another concept in the lower bounds. This situation generally suggests a missing hierarchical relation between concepts in the upper bounds (or in the lower bounds). For instance, in the lower bounds of the SNOMED

CT non-lattice subgraph in Fig. 5.5a, *duodenal, ulcer, with, perforation, and, obstruction* is contained in *chronic, duodenal, ulcer, with, perforation, and, obstruction*. Here, there is a missing hierarchical relation between concepts in the lower bounds because "*Chronic duodenal ulcer with perforation AND obstruction*" is more specific than "*Duodenal ulcer with perforation AND obstruction*." Of note, for this pattern, we specifically excluded non-lattice subgraphs with concepts that contain negation words such as *not, no, without, absence,* and *except*, because a missing hierarchical relation would be wrongly suggested between the concept with the negation and the same concept without negation. For example, the set of words for the concept "*Anemia during pregnancy—baby not yet delivered*" contains that of the concept "*Anemia during pregnancy—baby delivered as a subset*," but the two concepts are obviously not hierarchically related. Figure 5.6a contains a NCIt non-lattice subgraph exhibiting the containment pattern suggesting the missing hierarchical relation "*Stage III Nasopharyngeal Carcinoma AJCC v6*" is-a "*Stage III Nasopharyngeal Carcinoma*."

Fig. 5.5 a—A non-lattice subgraph exhibiting the Containment pattern in SNOMED CT. **b**—Suggested remediation for **a**. The suggested missing hierarchical relation is in red

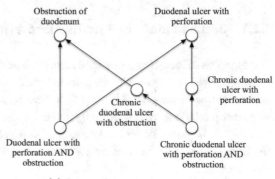

(a) **Pattern Containment - SNOMED CT**

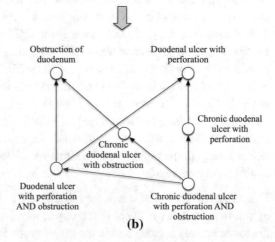

(b)

Fig. 5.6 a—A non-lattice subgraph exhibiting the Containment pattern in NCIt. **b**—Suggested remediation for **a**. The suggested missing hierarchical relation is in red

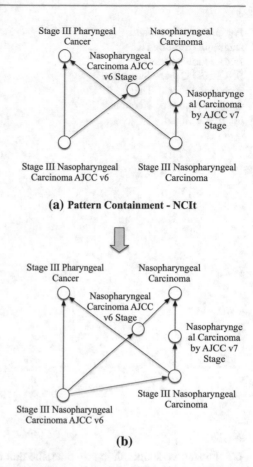

(a) Pattern Containment - NCIt

(b)

Intersection The intersection of sets of words for concepts in the lower bounds is equal to the set of words for some concept in the upper bounds. This situation generally suggests a missing hierarchical relation between concepts in the upper bounds. For example, in the SNOMED CT non-lattice subgraph Fig. 5.7a, the intersection of *irritable, bowel, syndrome, variant, of, childhood* and *irritable, bowel, syndrome, with, diarrhea* is *irritable, bowel, syndrome*, which is equal to the set of words for the concept *Irritable bowel syndrome* in the upper bounds. Here, there is a missing hierarchical relation between concepts in the upper bounds, because "*Irritable bowel syndrome*" is more specific than "*Disorder of colon.*" Similarly, Fig. 5.8a shows a NCIt non-lattice subgraph with the Intersection pattern indicating a missing hierarchical relation between the upper bound concepts "*Splenic Lymphoblastic Lymphoma*" and "*Aggressive Non-Hodgkin Lymphoma.*"

Union The union of the sets of words for concepts in the upper bounds is equal to the set of words for some concept in the lower bounds. This situation generally suggests a missing hierarchical relation between concepts in the lower bounds. For instance, in the SNOMED

Fig. 5.7 a—A non-lattice
subgraph exhibiting the
Intersection pattern in
SNOMED CT. **b**—Suggested
remediation for **a**. The
suggested missing hierarchical
relation is in red

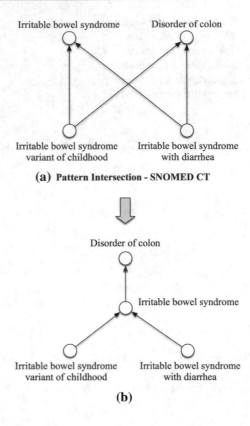

CT non-lattice subgraph in Fig. 5.9a, the union of *epithelial, neoplasm, of, skin* and *malignant, neoplasm, of, skin* is *malignant, epithelial, neoplasm, of, skin*, which is equal to the set of words for the concept "*Malignant epithelial neoplasm of skin*" in the lower bounds. Here, there is a missing hierarchical relation between concepts in the lower bounds, because "*Squamous cell carcinoma of skin*" is more specific than "*Malignant epithelial neoplasm of skin*." Likewise, Fig. 5.10a shows an NCIt non-lattice subgraph exhibiting Union pattern which suggests a missing hierarchical relation between the concepts "*Childhood Testicular Yolk Sac Tumor*" and "*Malignant Testicular Non-Seminomatous Germ Cell Tumor*."

Union-Intersection The union of the sets of words for concepts in the upper bounds is equal to the intersection of sets of words for concepts in the lower bounds. This situation generally suggests a missing intermediary concept between the upper bounds and the lower bounds. For instance, in the SNOMED CT non-lattice subgraph in Fig. 5.11a, the union of *neoplasm, right, upper, lobe, of, lung* and *malignant, neoplasm, upper, lobe, of, lung* is *malignant, neoplasm, right, upper, lobe, of, lung*, which is equal to the intersection of *secondary, malignant, neoplasm, right, upper, lobe, of, lung* and *primary, malignant, neoplasm, right, upper, lobe, of, lung*. Here, there is a missing concept, "*Malignant neoplasm*

Fig. 5.8 a—A non-lattice
subgraph exhibiting the
Intersection pattern in NCIt.
b—Suggested remediation for
a. The suggested missing
hierarchical relation is in red

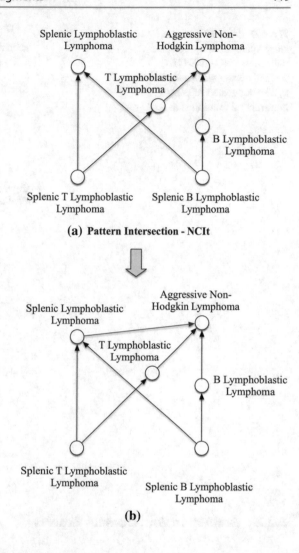

(a) **Pattern Intersection - NCIt**

(b)

of right upper lobe of lung," representing the features common to the two concepts in the
lower bounds ("*Primary malignant neoplasm of right upper lobe of lung*" and "*Secondary
malignant neoplasm of right upper lobe of lung*"), inherited from both concepts in the upper
bounds ("*Malignant neoplasm of upper lobe of lung*" and "*Neoplasm of right upper lobe of
lung*"). Similarly, Fig. 5.12a shows an NCIt non-lattice subgraph with the Union-Intersection
pattern indicating the missing concept "*Localized Adult Liver Carcinoma*.".

Fig. 5.9 a—A non-lattice subgraph exhibiting the Union pattern in SNOMED CT. **b**—Suggested remediation for **a**. The suggested missing hierarchical relation is in red

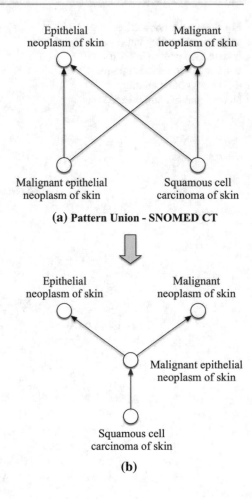

(a) Pattern Union - SNOMED CT

(b)

5.2.2   Evaluation with Domain Experts

To assess the effectiveness of our method in identifying real errors, we focused on small non-lattice subgraphs (size 4, 5, or 6) following any of the four lexical patterns. Evaluation samples were picked as follows for each ontology.

SNOMED CT
A random sample of 100 small subgraphs was selected from the two largest subhierarchies of SNOMED CT: *Clinical finding* and *Procedure*. The sample non-lattice subgraphs were rendered in Scalable Vector Graphics (SVGs) to facilitate visualization and evaluation by experts.

Fig. 5.10 a—A non-lattice subgraph exhibiting the Union pattern in NCIt. **b**—Suggested remediation for **a**. The suggested missing hierarchical relation is in red

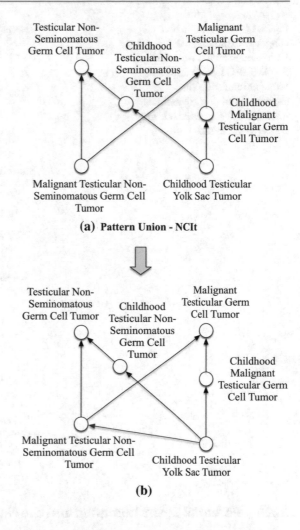

(a) **Pattern Union - NCIt**

(b)

To minimize the time and effort needed by the experts to review the subgraphs, we eliminated the most complex cases (e.g., subgraphs with multiple problems), as well as cases that are known issues. For example, the triaged subgraphs include those with terms containing AND/OR, which are progressively being eliminated in newer versions.

NCIt

A random sample of 45 non-lattice subgraphs was picked, and the non-lattice subgraphs as well as remediations were rendered in scalable vector graphics and provided to experts for evaluation.

Fig. 5.11 a—A non-lattice subgraph exhibiting the Union-Intersection pattern in SNOMED CT. **b**—Suggested remediation for **a**. The suggested missing hierarchical relations and suggested missing concepts are in red

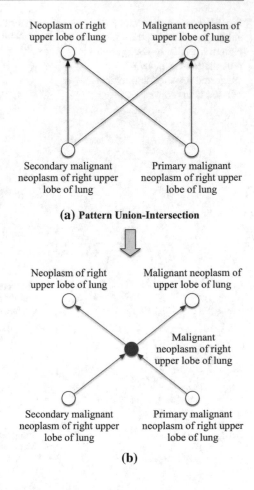

(a) Pattern Union-Intersection

(b)

5.2.3   Potential Errors Identified and the Findings of the Evaluation

From the September 2015 version of the SNOMED CT (U.S. edition), we identified 171,011 non-lattice subgraphs, of which 6,801 were found exhibiting any of the four lexical patterns. Among these, 2,046 were found to be small (sizes of 4, 5, and 6). The Intersection pattern accounted for the largest proportion (1,085) while Containment, Union, and Union-Intersection accounted for 736; 164; and 61, respectively.

On the other hand, from the 16.12d version of NCIt, we extracted a total of 8,143 non-lattice subgraphs among which 739 exhibited any of the lexical patterns. Out of the 739 non-lattice subgraphs 313 were found to be small. The Intersection pattern accounted for the largest proportion for NCIt as well (190). The containment, Union, and Union-Intersection patterns accounted for 114; 7; and 2, respectively.

Fig. 5.12 a—A non-lattice subgraph exhibiting the Union-Intersection pattern in NCIt. **b**—Suggested remediation for **a**. The suggested missing hierarchical relations and suggested missing concepts are in red

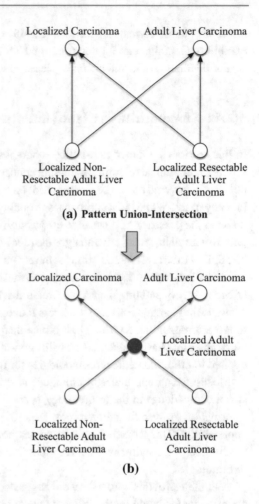

(a) **Pattern Union-Intersection**

(b)

Evaluation

SNOMED Of 100 subgraphs randomly selected, 37 exhibited the Containment pattern, 46 the Intersection pattern, 13 the Union pattern, and 4 the Union-Intersection pattern. Of the 100 non-lattice subgraphs, 59 were triaged for review by the medical experts. In each case, the experts confirmed the existence of an error. Therefore, the error rate among the 100 subgraphs is at least 59%. Among the 59 erroneous subgraphs examined, 34 exhibited a Containment pattern, 14 an Intersection pattern, 8 a Union pattern, and 3 a Union-Intersection pattern.

NCIt The 45 non-lattice subgraphs in the evaluation sample contained 19 exhibiting Containment, 22 exhibiting Intersection, 3 exhibiting Union and 1 exhibiting Union-Intersection. Of the 45 non-lattice subgraphs evaluated by domain experts, 29 were verified to contain errors and make correct suggestions ($29/45 = 64.44\%$). Among these 29 cases, 16 were exhibiting Containment, 9 Intersection, 3 Union, and 1 Union-Intersection.

For detailed results and analysis, please see [98, 99].

5.2.4 Summarization of the Findings

In this section, we mined non-lattice subgraphs exhibiting four lexical patterns to uncover missing hierarchical relations or missing concepts in SNOMED CT and NCIt. Our approach not only uncovered novel (i.e., unreported) errors but also suggested appropriate remediation in many cases. While most approaches to quality assurance of biomedical ontologies merely indicate the presence of a possible error, our hybrid approach overlays lexical information onto structural information to analyze the precise nature of the error and propose a correction. The ability to suggest remediation for the errors we identify, sets us apart from other methods and will likely drive adoption. Focusing on non-lattice subgraphs of smaller size provides an effective way of auditing hierarchical relations. Not only is it easier for experts to review and examine these graphs, but also the errors found in small graphs are mechanically propagated to larger graphs. Since virtually all biomedical ontologies are organized into subsumption hierarchies and have concept names, this non-lattice-based approach can be generalized and applied to other biomedical terminologies for quality assurance purposes.

Most existing approaches to biomedical quality assurance typically take advantage of specific knowledge in the terminology, such as lexical information [100–102] or structural information on specific subhierarchy, [88, 103–106] but have limitations in scalability and applicability. This work not only leverages both structural and lexical information and is not limited to a specific subhierarchy, but it is also scalable and widely applicable to other terminologies.

A limitation of this work is that our suggested remediation (e.g., to add missing hierarchical relations) is based on the inferred concept hierarchy of SNOMED CT and NCIt. Since this hierarchy is produced by a description logic classifier based on the logical definitions for the concepts, a more meaningful remediation would be to modify the logical definitions, so that the appropriate hierarchy can be inferred.

Conclusion: In this section, we introduced a novel structural-lexical approach leveraging non-lattice subgraphs and lexical information in concept names for detecting missing hierarchical relations or missing concepts in the SNOMED CT and NCIt. This approach differs from other quality assurance methods in that we also suggest remediation for the errors identified. We showed that identifying and analyzing small non-lattice subgraphs in both SNOMED CT and NCIt with lexical patterns is a simple and effective quality assurance technique.

5.3 Enriched Lexical Attributes in Non-lattices

In this section, we introduce a structural-lexical approach for auditing SNOMED CT using a combination of non-lattice subgraphs of the underlying hierarchical relations and enriched lexical attributes of fully specified concept names. This approach takes advantage of the rich lexical information contained in the ancestors of each concept in non-lattice subgraphs to facilitate the auditing process. Our goal is to develop a scalable and effective approach that automatically identifies missing *is-a* relations with high precision. A secondary goal is to uncover related incorrect *is-a* relations in the subgraphs.

5.3.1 The Steps of the Enriched Lexical Attributes Approach

We use the September 2017 release of SNOMED CT (US edition) in this approach. We extract all the non-lattice subgraphs in SNOMED CT. We enrich the lexical attributes of concepts in non-lattice subgraphs, identify missing hierarchical *is-a* relations between concepts based on the enriched lexical attributes. Clinical experts evaluate a random sample of suggested missing *is-a* relations to verify missing *is-a* relations and incorrect *is-a* relations.

Algorithm 1: Pseudocode for identifying missing *is-a* relations for a non-lattice subgraph based on enriched lexical attributes.

Input: A non-lattice subgraph G consisting of concepts and *is-a* relations
Output: Reclassified *is-a* relations
1 **if** *the fully specified name of a concept in G contains stop word(s) or antonyms* **then**
2 | stop here;
3 **else**
4 | continue;
5 **end**
6 Compute the transitive closure of the *is-a* relations in G;
7 Derive term pairs based on the transitive closure and fully specified names of the concepts in G;
8 **for** *each concept c in G* **do**
9 | Initialize a set L_c of lexical attributes for c using its fully specified name;
10 | Enrich L_c by leveraging the lexical attributes of c's ancestors;
11 | Enrich L_c by the derived term pairs;
12 **end**
13 **for** *each concept c_1 in G* **do**
14 | **for** *each concept c_2 in G* **do**
15 | | **if** $c_1 \neq c_2$ *and* $L_{c_1} \subseteq L_{c_2}$ **then**
16 | | | Suggest c_2 *is-a* c_1;
17 | **end**
18 **end**
19 Reduce the resulted *is-a* relations to direct *is-a* relations;

Algorithm 1 presents the pseudocode for identifying missing *is-a* relations for a given non-lattice subgraph based on enriched lexical attributes. The algorithm mainly consists of three steps: detection of stop words and antonyms (lines 1–5), construction of enriched lexical attributes (lines 6–12), and identification of missing *is-a* relations (lines 13–19). We describe these steps in detail and provide illustrative examples.

Detection of Stop Words and Antonyms

Since the lexical attributes of the concept "*Fetal hypertrophic cardiomyopathy due to maternal diabetes mellitus*" contain that of the concept "*Diabetes mellitus*," the relation "*Fetal hypertrophic cardiomyopathy due to maternal diabetes mellitus*" *is-a* "*Diabetes mellitus*" would be incorrectly generated. Similarly, "*Periostitis without osteomyelitis*" *is-a* "*Osteomyelitis*" would be incorrectly generated. Along the same lines, the concept "*Open reduction of closed sacral fracture*" contains antonyms "open" and "closed," and the concept "*Acute on chronic endometritis disorder*" contain antonyms "acute" and "chronic." Ignoring terms that contains antonyms prevents us from suggesting wrong relations, for example, between "*Open reduction of closed sacral fracture*" and "*Open reduction of open sacral fracture*." To prevent such issues, we exclude from processing those terms containing words, such as "due to" and "without." More generally, we extend this measure to a list of stop words and antonyms.

We consider the following as stop words: "and," "or," "and/or," "no," "not," "without," "due to," "secondary to," "except," "by," "after," "co-occurrent," "bilateral," "examination," "able," "amputation,""removal," "replacement," "resection," "excision." For antonyms, we rely on a list of pairs of antonyms from WordNet [107, 108], including ("anterior," "posterior"), ("chronic," "acute"), ("open," "closed"), ("positive," "negative"), ("high," "low"), ("benign," "malignant"), ("right," "left"), ("simple," "compound").

Given a non-lattice subgraph G, we detect if any concept in G contains stop word(s) and antonyms, which are prone to generate incorrect *is-a* relations using lexical attributes in practice. If stop word(s) or antonyms are detected, we discontinue the investigation of the non-lattice subgraph (i.e., stop the process of identifying missing *is-a* relations for G).

Construction of Enriched Lexical Attributes

Given a non-lattice subgraph G, we construct an enriched set of lexical attributes for each concept in G by leveraging three sources. The first source is the fully specified name of the concept itself, i.e., its own lexical attributes; the second source is the fully specified names of the concept's ancestors within the subgraph, i.e., often more generic words compared to the attributes of the concept itself; and the third source is a set of derived term pairs intended to capture hypernymy relations between individual words from hierarchically related concepts in the non-lattice subgraph.

To obtain the second source, we compute the transitive closure of the *is-a* relations in G, denoted by $T = \{(d, a)|$ concept a is an ancestor of concept d and $a \in G\}$. To obtain the third source, for each concept pair (d, a) in T, assuming W_d and W_a represent the sets of words contained in the concepts d and a, respectively; if $W_d \cap W_a \neq \emptyset$,

$W_d - (W_d \cap W_a) \neq \emptyset$, and $W_a - (W_d \cap W_a) \neq \emptyset$, we obtain a derived term pair $\left(W_d - (W_d \cap W_a), W_a - (W_d \cap W_a)\right)$. Take the concept pair (*"Fracture subluxation of perilunate joint,"* *"Fracture dislocation of perilunate joint"*) as an example. We have W_d={fracture, subluxation, of, perilunate, joint} and W_a={fracture, dislocation, of, perilunate, joint}, and thus $W_d \cap W_a$={fracture, of, perilunate, joint}, from which we derive the term pair ("subluxation," "dislocation"). This derived term pair captures the fact that dislocation is a hypernym of (i.e., is more generic than) subluxation.

Leveraging the three sources, we build an enriched set of lexical attributes (in lowercase) for each concept c in G as follows.

1. We initialize a set L_c of lexical attributes using the set of words contained in the fully specified name of c.
2. For each ancestor a of c within G, we enrich L_c by adding the set of words contained in the fully specified name of a.
3. For any derived term pair (p_1, p_2), if the term p_1 is contained in the fully specified name of c, then we further enrich L_c by adding the set of words in the term p_2.

We illustrate the process of constructing enriched lexical attributes using the non-lattice subgraph shown in Fig. 5.13a. This non-lattice subgraph consists of 6 concepts (numbered in circles). The initialized sets of lexical attributes using the fully specified names of the six concepts are:

$L_1 = $ {superficial, injury},
$L_2 = $ {injury, of, lower, extremity},
$L_3 = $ {traumatic, blister, of, lower, limb},
$L_4 = $ {friction, blisters, of, the, skin},
$L_5 = $ {superficial, injury, of, lower, limb},
$L_6 = $ {superficial, traumatic, blister, of, lower, limb}.

Leveraging the ancestors' lexical attributes results in the following enriched sets (with newly added lexical attributes *italicized*):

$L_1 = $ {superficial, injury},
$L_2 = $ {injury, of, lower, extremity},
$L_3 = $ {traumatic, blister, of, lower, limb, *injury, extremity*},
$L_4 = $ {friction, blisters, of, the, skin, *superficial, injury*},
$L_5 = $ {superficial, injury, of, lower, limb, *extremity*},
$L_6 = $ {superficial, traumatic, blister, of, lower, limb, *injury, extremity, friction, blisters, the, skin*}.

Leveraging the derived term pairs results in the same sets of lexical attributes (i.e., no additional lexical attributes are added for the concepts).

Figure 5.14a shows another example of a non-lattice subgraph. The initial sets of lexical attributes using the fully specified names of the six concepts are:

Fig. 5.13 An example of a non-lattice subgraph of size 6 in the *Clinical finding* sub-hierarchy, as well as the resulted subgraph after adding a missing *is-a* relation (red link): *"Superficial traumatic blister of lower limb" is-a "Superficial injury of lower limb"*

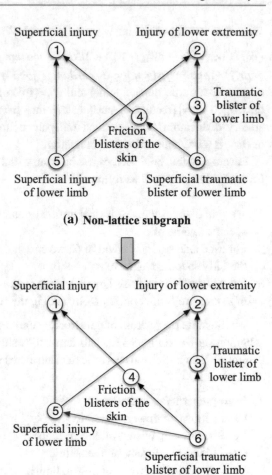

(a) **Non-lattice subgraph**

(b) **Subgraph with missing IS-A relation added**

$L_1 = \{$fracture, dislocation, of, lunate$\}$,
$L_2 = \{$fracture, subluxation, of, wrist$\}$,
$L_3 = \{$fracture, subluxation, of, lunate$\}$,
$L_4 = \{$fracture, dislocation, of, perilunate, joint$\}$,
$L_5 = \{$open, fracture, subluxation, lunate$\}$,
$L_6 = \{$fracture, subluxation, of, perilunate, joint$\}$,

Leveraging the ancestors' lexical attributes results in the following enriched sets (with newly added lexical attributes *italicized*):

$L_1 = \{$fracture, dislocation, of, lunate$\}$,
$L_2 = \{$fracture, subluxation, of, wrist$\}$,
$L_3 = \{$fracture, subluxation, of, lunate, *wrist*$\}$,

Fig. 5.14 An example of a non-lattice subgraph of size 6 in the "Clinical finding" sub-hierarchy, as well as the resulted subgraph after adding a missing *is-a* relation (red link): "Fracture subluxation of lunate" *is-a* "Fracture dislocation of lunate

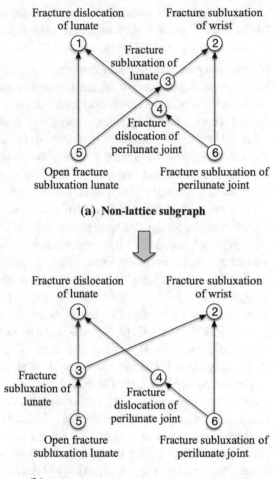

(a) **Non-lattice subgraph**

(b) **Subgraph with missing IS-A relation added**

$$L_4 = \{\text{fracture, dislocation, of, perilunate, joint, } \textit{lunate}\},$$
$$L_5 = \{\text{open, fracture, subluxation, lunate, } \textit{dislocation, of, wrist}\},$$
$$L_6 = \{\text{fracture, subluxation, of, perilunate, joint, } \textit{dislocation, lunate, wrist}\}.$$

Leveraging the derived term pairs results in the following final sets of lexical attributes (with newly added lexical attributes *italicized*):

$$L_1 = \{\text{fracture, dislocation, of, lunate}\},$$
$$L_2 = \{\text{fracture, subluxation, of, wrist, } \textit{dislocation}\},$$
$$L_3 = \{\text{fracture, subluxation, of, lunate, wrist, } \textit{dislocation}\},$$
$$L_4 = \{\text{fracture, dislocation, of, perilunate, joint, lunate}\},$$
$$L_5 = \{\text{open, fracture, subluxation, lunate, dislocation, of, wrist}\},$$
$$L_6 = \{\text{fracture, subluxation, of, perilunate, joint, dislocation, lunate, wrist}\}.$$

Note that the enrichment of L_2 and L_3 is due to the derived term pair ("subluxation," "dislocation"), which is obtained by the concept pair $(6, 4)$ in the transitive closure, that is, ("*Fracture subluxation of perilunate joint*," "*Fracture dislocation of perilunate joint*").

Identification of Missing is-a Relations

We compute all possible *is-a* relations between concepts in a given non-lattice subgraph G using the enriched lexical attributes for each concept (L_{c_i}). For any two concepts c_1 and c_2, if L_{c_1} is a proper subset of L_{c_2}, then we suggest c_2 is more specific than c_1 (or c_2 *is-a* c_1). Then we further reduce the computed *is-a* relations to direct *is-a* relations to eliminate relations that can be inferred from other relations. We compare the set of relations obtained from enriched lexical attributes of concepts in non-lattice subgraphs to the *is-a* relations present in the inferred hierarchy of SNOMED CT. The relations obtained through our approach, but not present in SNOMED CT, are considered missing relations.

For example, for the concepts numbered 5 and 6 in Fig. 5.13a, $L_5 = \{$superficial, injury, of, lower, limb, extremity$\}$ is a proper subset of $L_6 = \{$superficial, traumatic, blister, of, lower, limb, injury, extremity, friction, blisters, the, skin$\}$, thus we suggest concept 6 is more specific than concept 5, that is, "*Superficial traumatic blister of lower limb*" *is-a* "*Superficial injury of lower limb*" (see the red link in Fig. 5.13b). Computing all *is-a* relations in the graph in Fig. 5.13a results in the following set of *is-a* relations: $\{(4, 1), (5, 1), (6, 1), (3, 2), (5, 2), (6, 2), (6, 3), (6, 4), (6, 5)\}$, which can be further reduced to direct relations: $\{(4, 1), (5, 1), (3, 2), (5, 2), (6, 3), (6, 4), (6, 5)\}$. Here $(6, 5)$ is the newly identified relation, because all the others already exist in the original non-lattice subgraph.

For the concepts 1 and 3 in Fig. 5.14a, $L_1 = \{$fracture, dislocation, of, lunate$\}$ is a proper subset of $L_3 = \{$fracture, subluxation, of, lunate, wrist, dislocation$\}$, thus we suggest concept 3 is more specific than concept 1, that is, "*Fracture subluxation of lunate*" *is-a* "*Fracture dislocation of lunate*" (see the red link in Fig. 5.14b). Here $(3, 1)$ is a newly identified relation. Among the existing relations, our method also identifies $(3, 2)$, since $L_2 = \{$fracture, subluxation, of, wrist, dislocation$\}$ is a proper subset of $L_3 = \{$fracture, subluxation, of, lunate, wrist, dislocation$\}$.

Evaluation

We focus on small non-lattice subgraphs (of size 4, 5, and 6) to evaluate the effectiveness of our approach to suggesting missing *is-a* relations and revealing incorrect *is-a* relations in SNOMED CT. The rationale for focusing on non-lattice subgraphs of smaller size is twofold: one is that it is easier for experts to review these subgraphs, the other is that the errors found in small subgraphs are often also contained in larger subgraphs (as discussed in Sect. 5.2).

We selected a random sample of 200 non-lattice subgraphs from *Clinical finding* and *Procedure*, the two largest sub-hierarchies of SNOMED CT. The 200 subgraphs (223 *is-a* instances) were split into two sample sets (125 subgraphs each), with a shared common subset of 50 subgraphs (56 *is-a* instances). Two clinical experts independently reviewed the two sample sets with suggested missing *is-a* relations. For the commonly evaluated 50 subgraphs, differences in evaluation results were reconciled by discussion.

For the suggestions that were found incorrect by a clinical expert, we further reviewed the existing *is-a* relations in the original non-lattice subgraphs that were used to generate the suggestions. This is because the identification of a missing *is-a* relation can be due to the presence of an erroneous *is-a* relation in the subgraph. If the clinical expert also disagrees with the existing *is-a* relation, then this relation is identified as an incorrect *is-a* relation in SNOMED CT (source error). For instance, from the non-lattice subgraph in Fig. 5.14a, we also suggest that concept 6 is more specific than concept 3, that is, "*Fracture subluxation of perilunate joint*" *is-a* "*Fracture subluxation of lunate*." However, this invalid suggestion is derived in part from the existing relation (4, 1): "*Fracture dislocation of perilunate joint*" *is-a* "*Fracture dislocation of lunate*." Since perilunate dislocation is distinct from lunate dislocation, the existing relation is invalid in the first place. Therefore, although the missing *is-a* relation we identified is a false positive, our analysis of the non-lattice subgraph in Fig. 5.14a reveals an incorrect is-a relation (4, 1).

5.3.2   Overall Results and Evaluation

Non-lattice Subgraphs

A total of 195,121 non-lattice subgraphs were extracted. Among these, our approach based on enriched lexical attributes of the non-lattice subgraphs identified 14,380 subgraphs containing missing *is-a* relations. There were a total of 1,474 small non-lattice subgraphs (size of 4, 5, and 6).

Overall, the 14,380 non-lattice subgraphs contained a total of 41,357 missing *is-a* relations. The 1,474 small non-lattice subgraphs contained a total of 1,629 missing *is-a* relations. It is worth noting that a non-lattice subgraph may contain more than one missing *is-a* relations. Therefore, the number of missing *is-a* relations suggested was larger than the number of non-lattice subgraphs.

Evaluation

Of the 200 subgraphs randomly selected from 937 small non-lattice subgraphs in the two largest sub-hierarchies, 139 were in the *Clinical finding* sub-hierarchy, and 61 in the *Procedure* sub-hierarchy. Of the 200 subgraphs, 32 were of size 4, 86 of size 5, and 82 of size 6.

The 200 subgraphs contain a total of 223 missing *is-a* relations. Upon review, two clinical experts concluded that 185 (82.96%) missing *is-a* relations are valid. For the invalid suggestions (false positives for suggested missing *is-a* relations), the experts further examined the existing *is-a* relations in SNOMED CT which were used for generating the suggestions, and identified 22 existing *is-a* relations to be incorrect (confirmed source errors), beyond those that were evaluated.

A total of 56 missing *is-a* relations within the 50 non-lattice subgraphs were evaluated by both evaluators. The two evaluators initially had agreed on 46 out of 56 (82.14%) of the cases. After reconciliation, all the discrepancies were resolved except 1 case (no agreement was

Fig. 5.15 A non-lattice subgraph of size 4 and the resulted subgraph after adding a missing *is-a* relations (red link): *"Renal angle tenderness" is-a "Renal pain"*

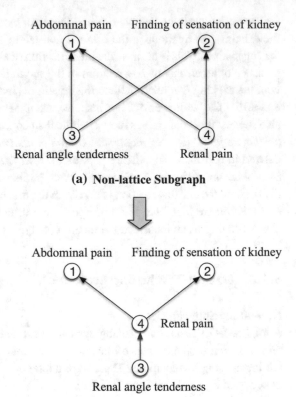

(a) **Non-lattice Subgraph**

(b) **Subgraph with missing IS-A relation added**

reached for this case). In addition, 3 cases were flagged as potentially contentious although an agreement was reached. The invalid suggestions further revealed 4 incorrect *is-a* relations in SNOMED CT as the source of error.

Figure 5.15 shows the non-lattice subgraph with the missing relation *"Renal angle tenderness" is-a "Renal pain."*

Figure 5.16 shows the non-lattice subgraph exhibiting the incorrect *is-a* relation: *"Congenital cyst of posterior segment of eye" is-a "Disorder of anterior segment of eye"* (see the red cross), which leads to the incorrect suggestion *"Congenital cyst of posterior segment of eye" is-a "Congenital anomaly of anterior segment of eye"* using our approach.

For detailed results, analysis, and explanations, please see [109–111].

Fig. 5.16 Non-lattice subgraph exhibiting an **incorrect** *is-a* relation (source error) in SNOMED CT (red cross): "*Congenital cyst of posterior segment of eye*" *is-a* "*Disorder of anterior segment of eye*

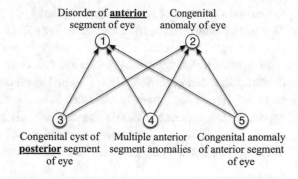

5.3.3   Further Analysis of the Approach and the Results

False Positives and Intricate Cases

Even though our hybrid approach was aimed at identifying missing hierarchical relations with high precision, false positives could not be completely eliminated. In some cases, the concepts contain implicit knowledge and have misleading surface forms. For example, our method suggests that "*Infection of toe web*" *is-a* "*Infection of toe*," which is incorrect. Toe web refers to the interdigital space of foot and is not a part of toe. Another example is that our method recommends "*Humerus head juvenile osteochondritis*" as a subclass of "*Humerus juvenile osteochondritis*," based on the observation that both concepts denote a form of humerus osteochondritis, and that one of them is further specified as juvenile. However, the juvenile form affects the humerus head, while the more general form affects the epicondyle, at the other extremity of the bone. In both cases, lexical similarity between the two terms is responsible for the false positives.

Similarly, our method suggests an *is-a* relation between the disorder concepts "*Budd-Chiari syndrome*" and "*Hepatic vein thrombosis.*" However, this relation does not always stand, since Budd-Chiari syndrome can also be due to compression (not thrombosis) of the hepatic veins. Here, the presence of an erroneous *is-a* relation in SNOMED CT between "*Budd-Chiari syndrome*" and "*Thrombosis of vein of trunk*" contributed to the wrongful suggestion.

Sometimes part-whole relationships may give opposite conclusions in different contexts. For example, one of the false positives is the suggestion that "*Does use the elements of language*" *is-a* "*Does use language.*" Since using elements of a language is not the same as the ability to use the language, this *is-a* relation is incorrect. However, if a subject has "*Difficulty using the elements of language*," then the subject must have "*Difficulty using [the] language.*" This would result in a true positive for our method.

Of note, during the evaluation, we observed a few cases for which it was difficult to determine whether the suggested missing *is-a* relation was correct or not. However, in the vast majority of cases, the experts had no difficulty agreeing on whether the suggested *is-a* relations were true or false positives.

Enhanced Coverage of Non-lattice Subgraphs

This work builds on the work discussed in Sect. 5.2, in that both leverage non-lattice graph substructures. The distinction is the substantially larger number of non-lattice subgraphs that were covered by the approach presented in this section. Applying the approach discussed in Sect. 5.2, to the same SNOMED CT version (September 2017 US edition), only 2,124 of 14,380 non-lattice subgraphs identified in this work can be detected using the previous approach. This represents 85.23% increase in coverage. Among non-lattice subgraphs of size 4, 5, and 6, 77.61% were newly identified (1,144 out of 1,474). Therefore, our recommendation for ontology quality assurance would be to use both approaches.

Limitations

Despite the substantially increased coverage of non-lattice subgraphs, we are only able to cover 7.4% of all non-lattice subgraphs. Identifying new lexical patterns among the non-lattice subgraphs remains an active topic for research.

Automatic change suggestion for identified errors is a unique feature of our approach. However, the change suggestions pertain to the inferred hierarchy. Since this hierarchy is inferred by a description logic classifier based on the logical definitions of concepts, the only meaningful remediation would be to find the root cause and modify the logical definitions so that the appropriate hierarchy can be inferred. Identifying erroneous and missing axioms in logical definitions will be the object of future work.

Conclusion: This section introduced a novel approach to predicting missing *is-a* relations in SNOMED CT by combining non-lattice subgraphs and enriched lexical attributes of concepts. Our result of a 82.96% precision on the predicted missing relations demonstrates that leveraging enriched lexical attributes within non-lattice subgraphs is an effective approach for auditing SNOMED CT. Since a hierarchical substructure and lexical attributes of concepts are present in almost all biomedical ontologies, this method is generally applicable for ontology quality assurance purposes.

5.4   Hybrid Methods

In this section, we discuss a hybrid model in which role definitions of concepts in non-lattice subgraphs are harmonized with lexical features to assist with the subsumption checking of *is-a* relations between concept pairs.

Lexical Features and Role Definitions in Biomedical Ontologies

To automatically identify missing *is-a* relations, one commonly used approach is to find features to represent the meanings of concepts [112, 113] and check whether there exists any subsumption relation between the represented meanings. In biomedical ontologies, two important aspects can be utilized to represent the semantic meaning of a concept – lexical features and role definitions.

Though lexical features have been widely adopted to detect missing hierarchical relations in ontologies, in many cases, it is challenging to get the machine to catch the meanings and other details behind the words. Take concept "*Sarcoma*" in the NCI Thesaurus as an example. Purely from the concept name itself, the machine will not be able to know that this concept refers to a malignant neoplasm of the soft tissue or bone. In addition, concept names are defined manually by curators of biomedical ontologies, and inconsistencies may exist during the naming process, which may further affect the subsumption checking.

When it comes to role definitions, most modern ontologies provide formally defined role definitions (in a format of relations between concepts) to represent meanings of concepts. There are two types of relations involved in the role definition of a concept: hierarchical *is-a* relations and associative roles, where the *is-a* relations determine the concept's location in the hierarchy (e.g., its supertypes and its subtypes) and the associative roles are the role assertions that further define the concept. We denote the role definition of a concept as (*role, value*) pairs, where *value* refers to the target concept to which this concept connects through the *role*. Table 5.1 shows role definitions of concept "*Sarcoma*" in the NCI Thesaurus consisting of two *is-a* relations and 11 associative roles. For example, (*is-a, Malignant Neoplasm*) is an *is-a* relation while (*Disease_Has_Associated_Anatomic_Site*, *Connective and Soft Tissue*) is an associative role. These kinds of role definitions refine the meanings of concepts. However, role definitions are often incomplete making them impractical to be solely used in representing meanings of concepts. For instance, in 19.08d version of the NCI Thesaurus, only 17,052 out of 146,688 (11.62%) concepts are considered fully defined in role definition; and in 11/02/2019 release of the Gene Ontology, the number is 12,011 out of 44,650 (26.9%).

Table 5.1 The role definitions of concept "*Sarcoma*" (C9118) in NCI Thesaurus

Role	Value
is-a	Connective and Soft Tissue Neoplasm
is-a	Malignant Neoplasm
Disease_Has_Abnormal_Cell	Malignant Cell
Disease_Has_Abnormal_Cell	Neoplastic Cell
Disease_Excludes_Normal_Cell_Origin	Epithelial Cell
Disease_Excludes_Normal_Tissue_Origin	Epithelial Tissue
Disease_Has_Associated_Anatomic_Site	Connective and Soft Tissue
Disease_Has_Normal_Tissue_Origin	Connective and Soft Tissue
Disease_Excludes_Finding	Benign Cellular Infiltrate
Disease_Excludes_Finding	Indolent Clinical Course
Disease_Excludes_Finding	Intermediate Filaments Present
Disease_Excludes_Finding	Intracytoplasmic Eosinophilic Inclusion
Disease_Has_Finding	Malignant Cellular Infiltrate

5.4.1 Main Steps of the Hybrid Model

As discussed in Sects. 5.1, 5.2, and 5.3, non-lattice subgraphs in biomedical ontologies often reveal quality issues including missing *is-a* relations. Therefore, in this work, we focus on non-lattice subgraphs to detect missing *is-a* relations. To identify missing *is-a* relations in non-lattice subgraphs, we first find a proper way to represent the meanings of concepts, and then check whether there exists any subsumption relations between the represented meaning of unlinked concepts (i.e., not connected by *is-a* relations either directly or transitively) within non-lattice subgraphs.

There are mainly three steps: (1) compute non-lattice subgraphs and identify candidate pairs of concepts that are currently not linked by *is-a* relations; (2) for each concept, construct model that harmonizes role definitions, words, and roots of noun chunks within its concept name and its ancestor's names to represent its meanings; (3) perform subsumption checking for candidate pairs based on our hybrid model.

Computing Non-lattice Subgraphs and Generating Candidate Pairs
We leverage an efficient non-lattice extraction algorithm introduced in Sect. 4.3 to compute all the non-lattice subgraphs in the NCI Thesaurus. Then we identify potentially missing *is-a* relations between pairs of concepts (denoted as candidate pairs) which are currently not linked by *is-a* relations in the non-lattice subgraphs. Take the non-lattice subgraph shown in Fig. 5.17 as an example, ("*Non-Neoplastic Skin Disorder,*" "*Cutaneous Pseudolymphoma*") is a candidate pair and ("*Skin Disorder,*" "*Benign Lymphoproliferative Disorder*") is another.

Fig. 5.17 An example of non-lattice subgraphs in 19.08d version of NCI Thesaurus. Concepts are connected by *is-a* relations. The red dotted line shows a potential missing *is-a* relation between concepts "*Cutaneous Pseudolymphoma*" and "*Non-Neoplastic Skin Disorder*" identified by our method

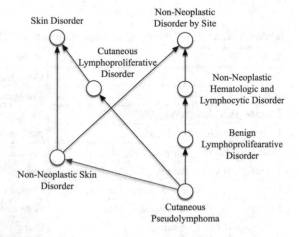

Modeling Concepts

In this work, we introduce a comprehensive semantic model which utilizes role definitions and lexical features to represent the meaning of concepts.

Given a concept C, its semantic model contains five parts $(C_{bow}, C_{ebow}, C_r, C_{er}, C_a)$:

1. bag-of-words C_{bow}, which includes words appearing in its preferred name;
2. enriched bag-of-words C_{ebow}, which includes words appearing in its preferred name and words in its ancestors' preferred names;
3. roots of noun chunks C_r, which includes roots of noun chunks in its preferred name;
4. enriched roots of noun chunks C_{er}, which includes roots of noun chunks in its preferred name and in its ancestors' preferred names; and
5. associative roles C_a.

Figure 5.18 shows the semantic models for concepts *"Cutaneous Pseudolymphoma"* and *"Non-Neoplastic Skin Disorder"* in the non-lattice subgraph shown in Fig. 5.17. Note that *is-a* relations in the role definitions are not included in the semantic model since our goal is to identify missing *is-a* relations. Alternatively, we use features inherited from concept's ancestor (i.e., C_{ebow} and C_{er}) to embody the *is-a* relations, which could gather more concept related information and thus help refine the meaning of concepts. We maintain both original lexical features (i.e., C_{bow} and C_r) and enriched ones (i.e., C_{ebow} and C_{er}) for performing subsumption testing later.

Lexical Features   The regular bag-of-words C_{bow} and enriched bag-of-words C_{ebow} could convey the meaning of a concept to some extent. However, there exist some words that may express different meanings depending on the contexts under which they appear. For example, word "erlotinib" in concept *"Erlotinib"* and in concept *"Erlotinib Hydrochloride"* convey different meanings – the former refers to the chemical item itself while the latter is used to describe word "hydrochloride." Therefore, even though both concepts contain the same word "erlotinib," it should be considered as a different lexical feature for each concept.

To handle such cases (i.e., noun used as a descriptive term), our idea is to leverage a technique in Natural Language Processing (NLP) called dependency parsing, which could extract the grammatical structure and relationships between words for a given phrase. For example, after parsing concept name *"Malignant Bladder Neoplasm,"* we can get "malignant bladder neoplasm" whole as a noun chunk. The word "malignant" is used to modify "neoplasm" in terms of the type (i.e., benign or malignant) while the word "bladder" is used to modify "neoplasm" in term of the location (i.e., anatomic site). In this work, besides bag-of-words C_{bow} (and enriched C_{ebow}), we also adopt roots of noun chunks C_r (and enriched C_{er}) as part of the lexical feature. Given a concept name, we use spaCy [114], an open-source library for NLP, to parse it and recognize the roots of noun chunks. In the previous example, "neoplasm" is denoted as a root of noun chunk since other words are used to modify it. By utilizing roots of noun chunks C_r, to some extent we could distinguish different meanings of a word in different context. In the concepts *"Erlotinib"* and *"Erlotinib Hydrochloride,"*

Cutaneous Pseudolymphoma (C62776)

Bag-of-Words	cutaneous, pseudolymphoma
Enriched Bag-of-Words	cutaneous, pseudolymphoma, benign, lymphoproliferative, disorder, skin, non-neoplastic
Roots of Noun Chunks	pseudolymphoma
Enriched Roots of Noun Chunks	pseudolymphoma, disorder
Associative Roles	(Disease_Has_Primary_Anatomic_Site, Skin), (Disease_Has_Finding, Perivascular Lymphocytic Infiltrate), (Disease_May_Have_Finding, Regression), (Disease_May_Have_Finding, Papular Lesion), (Disease_Has_Associated_Anatomic_Site, Skin), (Disease_Has_Associated_Anatomic_Site, Integumentary System), (Disease_Has_Associated_Anatomic_Site, Hematopoietic and Lymphatic System), (Disease_Has_Primary_Anatomic_Site, Lymphatic System), (Disease_Has_Primary_Anatomic_Site, Hematopoietic and Lymphatic System), (Disease_Has_Normal_Tissue_Origin, Lymphoid Tissue), (Disease_Has_Normal_Tissue_Origin, Hematopoietic and Lymphoid Tissue), (Disease_Has_Normal_Cell_Origin, Lymphocyte), (Disease_Has_Normal_Cell_Origin, Hematopoietic and Lymphoid Cell), (Disease_Has_Abnormal_Cell, Abnormal Lymphocyte), (Disease_Has_Finding, Non-Malignant Cellular Infiltrate), (Disease_Has_Finding, Cutaneous Involvement), (Disease_Excludes_Normal_Cell_Origin, Myeloid Cell), Disease_Excludes_Molecular_Abnormality, Clonal Antigen Receptor Gene Rearrangement)

Non-Neoplastic Skin Disorder (C27555)

Bag-of-Words	non-neoplastic, skin, disorder
Enriched Bag-of-Words	non-neoplastic, skin, disorder
Roots of Noun Chunks	disorder
Enriched Roots of Noun Chunks	disorder
Associative Roles	(Disease_Has_Associated_Anatomic_Site, Integumentary System), (Disease_Has_Primary_Anatomic_Site, Skin), (Disease_Has_Finding, Cutaneous Involvement)

Fig. 5.18 Semantic model of concepts "*Cutaneous Pseudolymphoma*" (C62776) and "*Non-Neoplastic Skin Disorder*" (C27555) which are contained in non-lattice subgraph shown in Fig. 5.17

word "erlotinib" will be taken as two different words – a root of noun chunk in the former concept, but a descriptive term (i.e., not a root of noun chunk) in the latter concept.

We also adopt a list of stop words that may distort the represented meanings of concepts. As mentioned in Sect. 5.4, concept names which contain "and" are often inconsistent with what they actually mean and their role definitions. For example, concept "*Lip **and** Oral Cavity Squamous Cell Carcinoma*" actually refers to a squamous cell carcinoma arising from the lip **or** the oral cavity. In this work, we do not perform subsumption testing for candidate pairs that include concepts whose C_{bow} contain any stop word. In addition, while generating enriched lexical features C_{ebow} and C_{er}, concepts will not inherit lexical features C_{bow} and C_r from their ancestors containing any stop word such that the stop words will not propagate. More specifically, as long as an ancestor contains a stop word, none of the ancestor's lexical features will be inherited. The list of stop words used in this step is the same as the one used in the lexical-based method discussed in Sect. 5.3.

In Fig. 5.18, it can be seen that concept "*Cutaneous Pseudolymphoma*" has two single words and inherits seven words from its ancestors such as "*Benign Lymphoproliferative Disorder*," "*Skin Disorder*" and "*Non-Neoplastic Disorder*," which enrich the meaning expressed by the concept. Also, word "pseudolymphoma" is recognized as the root of noun chunk "cutaneous pseudolymphoma." Concept "*Cutaneous Pseudolymphoma*" also inherits another root of noun chunk "disorder" from its ancestor "*Benign Lymphoproliferative Disorder*." Note that another ancestor of concept "*Cutaneous Pseudolymphoma*" is "*Non-Neoplastic Hematologic and Lymphocytic Disorder*," which contains the stop word "and." Hence, C_{bow} and C_r of this ancestor are not inherited.

Associative Roles In our model, we use associative roles C_a to collect and adjust the meaning of concepts which may not be fully expressed by lexical features, especially for concepts that are lexically similar but should not be linked by *is-a* relations. Consider the concepts "*Metastatic Malignant Neoplasm in the Pancreas*" and "*Metastatic Malignant Pancreatic Neoplasm*." If only lexical features are considered, the former concept's lexical features include all of the latter one's after the enrichment (e.g., "*Metastatic Malignant Neoplasm in the Pancreas*" inherits "pancreatic" from its ancestor "*Pancreatic Neoplasm*"). However, the former concept "*Metastatic Malignant Neoplasm in the Pancreas*" refers to a malignant neoplasm that has spread to the pancreas from another anatomic site, while "*metastatic malignant pancreatic neoplasm*" actually refers to a malignant neoplasm that arises from the pancreas and has metastasized to another anatomic site. Thus, there should not be any subsumption relation between these two concepts. However, the difference between the two concepts can not be caught purely from their lexical features. To compensate this, we adopt associative roles which usually contain information that are not included in the literal meanings. Consider the previous example, the former concept has an associative role (*Disease_Has_Metastatic_Anatomic_Site, Pancreas*), but the latter concept has role definition (*Disease_Excludes_Metastatic_Anatomic_Site, Pancreas*). Depending on the inclusion and exclusion of metastatic anatomic locations provided by the role definitions could easily distinguish these two concepts.

In this work, to gather as much information as possible, the associative roles we adopted for a concept are the inferred ones that include associative roles inherited from the concept's ancestors. For instance, in Fig. 5.18, concept "*Cutaneous Pseudolymphoma*" contains 18 associative roles (14 inherited from its ancestors), while concept "*Non-Neoplastic Skin Disorder*" contains three associative roles (two inherited from its ancestors).

Identifying Potentially Missing is-a Relations
As mentioned earlier, in this work, our task is to identify potentially missing *is-a* relations among candidate pairs – pairs of concepts that are not linked by *is-a* relations within non-lattice subgraphs. For each candidate pair (A, B), we perform a two-step subsumption checking to see if the meaning represented by the hybrid model of A is more detailed than B's (i.e., A *is-a* B), or vice versa (i.e., B *is-a* A).

In the first step, we perform a lexical-feature-based checking. We consider original lexical features (i.e., C_{bow}, C_r) as minimal satisfying features for a concept. In other words, if A's enriched lexical features (i.e., all meanings from lexical features that hold for A) satisfy B's original lexical features, we consider A is more detailed than B in terms of lexical features. Here, we do not consider enriched lexical features of B because A can then also inherit lexical features from B's ancestors if A becomes a subtype of B. As we represent lexical features of concepts as sets of words, we simply use set inclusion testing, that is, if A's enriched bag-of-words (i.e., A_{ebow}) is a superset of B's bag-of-words (i.e., B_{bow}) and A's enriched roots of noun chunks (i.e., A_{er}) is a superset of B's roots of noun chunks (i.e., B_r), then A is considered more detailed than B in lexical feature-wise.

In the second step, we perform a role-based checking. To do so, we require that each of the two concepts within a candidate pair should contain at least one associative role and associative roles of two concepts should not be totally identical (otherwise we can not decide which one is more detailed). Further, we check that for each associative role ($role_B$, $value_B$) of B, if there exists a corresponding role ($role_A$, $value_A$) of A such that $role_A$ and $role_B$ are the same and $value_B$ is the same or more general than $value_A$ (i.e., $value_B$ is an ancestor of $value_A$). If this is the case, then A is considered more detailed than B in terms of role definitions.

If A is more detailed than B in terms of both lexical features and role definitions, we consider "A is-a B" as a potentially missing is-a relation. For example, consider a candidate pair ("*Cutaneous Pseudolymphoma*," "*Non-Neoplastic Skin Disorder*") in Fig. 5.18. "*Cutaneous Pseudolymphoma*" is more detailed than "*Non-Neoplastic Skin Disorder*" in terms of lexical features because the enriched bag-of-words of "*Cutaneous Pseudolymphoma*," {cutaneous, pseudolymphoma, benign, lymphoproliferative, disorder, skin, non-neoplastic}, is a superset of bag-of-words of "*Non-Neoplastic Skin Disorder*," {non-neoplastic, skin, disorder}; and the enriched roots of noun chunks of "*Cutaneous Pseudolymphoma*," {pseudolymphoma, disorder}, is also a superset of roots of noun chunks of "*Non-Neoplastic Skin Disorder*," {disorder}. In addition, "*Cutaneous Pseudolymphoma*" is more detailed than "*Non-Neoplastic Skin Disorder*" in role definitions, since for each associative role of "*Non-Neoplastic Skin Disorder*," there is a corresponding role of "*Cutaneous Pseudolymphoma*" that is equivalent or more detailed. Therefore, our approach suggests "*Cutaneous Pseudolymphoma is-a Non-Neoplastic Skin Disorder*" as a potentially missing is-a relation. Note that this missing is-a relation has been confirmed by experts from NCI Enterprise Vocabulary Service (EVS) and included in the newer versions of the NCI Thesaurus.

In some cases, a potentially missing is-a relation detected could actually be a relation similar to an is-a relation, such as *part-of*. NCI Thesaurus provides associations (i.e., different things from role definitions) between concepts, such as *Has_Salt_Form*, *Has_Target*, *Has_Pharmaceutical_Transformation*, etc. We further utilize them to distinguish those like-is-a relations. Given a potentially missing is-a relation identified by our approach, if two concepts are already linked by any kind of these associations, then the missing is-a relation will be abandoned.

Another thing to consider is that due to the large size of some non-lattice subgraphs, there may exist an overlap between non-lattice subgraphs which may result in redundant missing *is-a* relations being suggested. For example, our approach may suggest "*A is-a B*" in one non-lattice subgraph and suggest "*A is-a C*" in another, while *B* is an ancestor of *C* in the current ontology (i.e., an existing *is-a* relation). In this case, "*A is-a B*" is considered redundant because it can be implied by the potentially missing *is-a* relation "*A is-a C*" and the existing relation "*C is-a B*." To improve the evaluation efficiency, we avoid unnecessary analyses on such redundant relations. More formally, a detected potentially missing *is-a* relation "*A is-a B*" is considered as redundant if it can be inferred by other missing or existing *is-a* relations.

5.4.2   Findings in NCI Thesaurus

We applied our enhanced hybrid approach to the NCI Thesaurus (19.08d inferred version [115]) for identifying potentially missing *is-a* relations. We briefly discuss our findings in the following sections. Please see [116, 117] for detailed results and analysis.

Non-lattice Subgraphs and Suggested is-a Relations
In total, 10,216 non-lattice subgraphs were obtained in 16 sub-hierarchies of the NCI Thesaurus. 55 non-redundant missing *is-a* relations were suggested for five sub-hierarchies.

Evaluation
For evaluation, we provided the NCI EVS domain experts, who manage the NCI Thesaurus, with 55 potentially missing *is-a* relations identified by our approach. 29 out of 55 were confirmed by EVS experts and have been incorporated in the newer version of the NCI Thesaurus. Valid missing *is-a* relations verified by EVS experts include "*Glycine Encephalopathy*" *is-a* "*Congenital Nervous System Disorder*" and "*Congenital Vena Cava Abnormality*" *is-a* "*Congenital Cardiovascular Abnormality*."

5.4.3   Further Analysis

False Positives
By reviewing invalid *is-a* relation suggestion by the approach, we identified two major causes for them.

The first cause is that the existence of erroneous *is-a* relations in NCI Thesaurus has led to invalid missing *is-a* suggestions. For example, our approach suggested "*Carcinosarcoma of the Mouse Prostate Gland*" *is-a* "*Carcinoma of the Mouse Prostate Gland*" mainly based on an existing *is-a* relation "*Carcinosarcoma of the Mouse Prostate Gland*" *is-a* "*Mouse Carcinoma*." However, as stated by EVS experts, "carcinosarcoma" is not a kind of "carcinoma." Thus, the existing *is-a* relation on which we rely to derive the missing *is-a* relation is incorrect, and it has been fixed by EVS experts in the newer release of the NCI Thesaurus. In total, 7 out of 26 false positive cases fall into this cause. In such cases, even though our suggestions of missing *is-a* relations were incorrect, they further revealed problems within the existing hierarchy of the NCI thesaurus that in turn help improve the quality of the NCI thesaurus.

Secondly, since we only adopted original lexical features (C_{bow}, C_r) for superconcepts during subsumption testing, the meanings beyond the original lexical features and logical definitions could lead incorrect missing *is-a* relations to be suggested. Consider the false positive "*Diffuse Pulmonary Lymphangiomatosis*" *is-a* "*Pulmonary Vascular Disorder*." The subconcept is a kind of "neoplasm," however, the superconcept has an ancestor "*Non-Neoplastic Lung Disorder*." Since a neoplasm could not be a subtype of a non-neoplastic disorder, this suggestion is invalid. Other similar cases include: "*Conjunctival Kaposi Sarcoma*" *is-a* "*Conjunctival Vascular Disorder*" and "*Retinal Hemangioma*" *is-a* "*Retinal Vascular Disorder*." Since meanings like "non-neoplastic" could be found in the enriched lexical features of superconcepts (i.e., inherited from ancestors), a natural question would be: Whether adopting enriched lexical features for both concepts within candidate pairs during lexical-based subsumption testing could improve the performance of our method?

To study this, we further utilized enriched lexical features of superconcept and subconcepts in lexical-based subsumption checking. Therefore, in order for an *is-a* relation to be suggested, the enriched lexical features of the subconcept now should also contain the original lexical features of the superconcept's ancestors. In total, 45 missing *is-a* relations were identified in this setting. The result was found to be a subset of our previous result. One exception is that a missing *is-a* relation was considered redundant but became non-redundant as some missing *is-a* relations are no longer included in the result. Since the *is-a* relation was redundant to a valid *is-a* relation, this *is-a* relation is also considered as valid. Among those 45 missing *is-a* relations, 29 were valid *is-a* relations, the number of true positives went down by 3 but the number of false positives went down by 7. We noticed that some false positives in the format of "neoplasm" *is-a* "non-neoplastic" still appeared in the result because the role definitions of the superconcepts are not sufficient (i.e., incompleteness). For example, "*Kidney Lymphangioma*" *is-a* "*Kidney Vascular Disorder*." The superconcept "*Kidney Vascular Disorder*" should be a "non-neoplastic" disorder, however, in the role definitions, none of its ancestors is "non-neoplastic" disorder and none of its associative roles indicates that it is not a kind of "neoplasm." Another example is "*Brain Astrocytoma*" *is-a* "*Brain Disorder*." Therefore, adopting enriched lexical features for both superconcept and subconcept during lexical-based subsumption checking could improve the performance, but only slightly due to the incompleteness of role definitions.

Limitations and Future Work

Although the results showed that our hybrid approach is promising in identifying missing *is-a* relations, there are several aspects that could be further improved.

In this approach, we directly used words in concepts names to form lexical features C_{bow} and C_{ebow}. Variants of the words (e.g., "disorder" and "disorders") that may be used to express the same meaning were not considered. As a result, some missing *is-a* relations may not be detected. Future work would be to perform normalization by stemming for concept names to identify more missing *is-a* relations.

In addition, missing *is-a* relations identified by our approach were from 184 out of 10,216 non-lattice subgraphs. New approaches are needed to further reveal potential quality issues in the remaining larger portion of non-lattice subgraphs in the NCI Thesaurus. Recent studies [113] have explored the feasibility of machine learning-based approaches to facilitate the identification of missing *is-a* relations in biomedical ontologies, indicating that further enhancement is still needed. In future work, we plan to explore how to adapt our hybrid model into embeddings for concepts and leverage machine learning techniques to uncover additional missing *is-a* relations.

Conclusion: In this section, we introduced a hybrid model that combines lexical features and role definitions of concepts to identify missing *is-a* relations within non-lattice subgraphs in the NCI Thesaurus. The results showed that our approach is capable of uncovering valid missing *is-a* relations. Further examination of false positives revealed erroneous existing *is-a* relations as well as incomplete concept definitions, which in turn also helped improve the quality of the NCI thesaurus.

Lexical Sequences and Patterns

In this chapter, we introduce lexical approaches to systematically detect potential *subtype* (or *is-a* relation) inconsistencies that can be generally applied to biomedical terminologies. These approaches utilize lexical information in concept names to uncover and suggest fixes to ontology defects.

6.1   Lexical-Based Inference

This approach leverages the names of pairs of concepts that are hierarchically linked and unlinked in a given terminology to derive potential inconsistencies, which may be indicative of missing subtype relations or incorrect existing subtype relations. We applied this approach to three terminologies: GO, NCIt, and SNOMED CT. To evaluate the effectiveness of this approach, we select a random sample of potential inconsistencies detected in GO, which were manually reviewed and validated by domain experts. We also performed a preliminary study on the extent to which external knowledge in the Unified Medical Language System (UMLS) can provide supporting evidence for validating the detected potential inconsistencies.

6.1.1   Inference Leveraging Lexical Sequences

Our lexical-based inference approach, aims at identifying potential subtype inconsistencies among concept-pairs in a given terminology. This approach leverages three intrinsic aspects of knowledge in the terminology: the names of concepts, the existing subtype relations, and the absent subtype relations.

© The Author(s), under exclusive license to Springer Nature Switzerland AG 2022
G.-Q. Zhang et al., *Formal Methods for the Analysis of Biomedical Ontologies*,
Synthesis Lectures on Data, Semantics, and Knowledge,
https://doi.org/10.1007/978-3-031-12131-9_6

Representation of Concept Names

The name of a concept in a terminology is used to unambiguously represent the semantic meaning of a concept. Given a terminology, we represent the name of each concept C as an ordered sequence of words $w_1 w_2 \ldots w_m$. For example, the name of a GO concept GO:0042317 (the unique identifier) is "*penicillin catabolic process*," and its sequence-of-words representation is [*penicillin, catabolic, process*].

Generation of Linked and Unlinked Concept-Pairs

A pair of concepts belonging to the same sub-hierarchy of a terminology, is defined as a *partial matching concept pair (PMCP)* with diff n, if the names of the two concepts have the same number of words and contain at least one word in common and n different words. We investigate $n = 1, 2, 3, 4, 5$ in this section. For instance, "*penicillin catabolic process*" (GO:0042317) and "*amine catabolic process*" (GO:0009310) is a PMCP with diff 1, because both of them are from the *biological process* sub-hierarchy of GO, contain two common words [*catabolic, process*], and differ in a single word—*penicillin* versus *amine*.

We classify PMCPs into two categories (linked and unlinked) as follows. If the two concepts in a PMCP have a subtype relation (either direct or indirect), then the PMCP is called a *linked PMCP*. If the two concepts in a PMCP do not have a subtype relation (neither direct nor indirect), then the PMCP is called an *unlinked PMCP*. Note that we pre-compute the transitive closure of the subtype relation (i.e., direct and indirect *is-a* relations) to decide whether a PMCP is linked or unlinked. That is, if two concepts of a PMCP are in the transitive closure, then the PMCP is linked; otherwise, it is unlinked.

Figure 6.1a presents an example of an unlinked PMCP with diff 1 in GO, where the two concepts "*siderophore metabolic process*" (GO:0009237) and "*peptide metabolic process*" (GO:0006518) differ in a single word—*siderophore* versus *peptide*.

Figure 6.2b presents an example of a linked PMCP with diff 2 in GO, where the two concepts "*regulation of synaptic metaplasticity*" (GO:0031916) and "*regulation of biological process*" (GO:0050789) differ in two words—*synaptic metaplasticity* versus *biological process*.

Generation of Linked and Unlinked Term-Pairs

For each PMCP (C_1, C_2), an *Inferred Term Pair (ITP)* can be derived as follows. Assume that $C_1 = w_{11} w_{12} \ldots w_{1m}$ and $C_2 = w_{21} w_{22} \ldots w_{2m}$ and there are n different words between C_1 and C_2: $w_{1i_1} w_{1i_2} \ldots w_{1i_n}$ versus $w_{2i_1} w_{2i_2} \ldots w_{2i_n}$, where $1 \leq i_j \leq m$ and $1 \leq j \leq n$. Then an ITP $(w_{1i_1} w_{1i_2} \ldots w_{1i_n}, w_{2i_1} w_{2i_2} \ldots w_{2i_n})$ is derived. In other words, the different words between the names of C_1 and C_2 derive an ITP. Note that we also require that the terms in difference cannot contain only numerals when generating ITPs.

We also classify ITPs into two categories (linked and unlinked) based on the PMCPs from which they are derived. An ITP derived from a linked PMCP is called a *linked ITP*. An ITP derived from an unlinked PMCP is called an *unlinked ITP*.

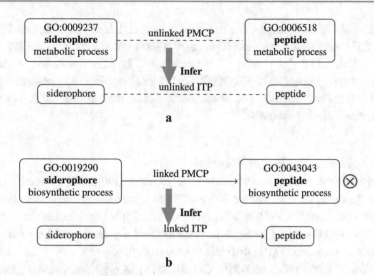

Fig. 6.1 a: Unlinked PMCP with diff 1 in GO and its unlinked ITP derived; **b**: Linked PMCP with diff 1 in GO and its linked ITP derived. This example reveals a potentially **incorrect existing subtype relation** in **b**, that is, "*siderophore biosynthetic process*" (GO:0019290) is not a subtype of "*peptide biosynthetic process*" (GO:0043043)

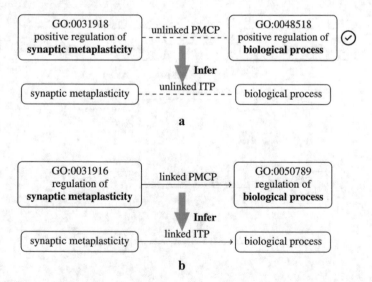

Fig. 6.2 a: An unlinked PMCP with diff 2 in GO and its unlinked ITP derived; **b**: A linked PMCP with diff 2 in GO and its linked ITP derived. This example reveals a potentially **missing subtype relation** in **a**, that is, "*positive regulation of synaptic metaplasticity*" (GO:0031918) *is-a* "*positive regulation of biological process*" (GO:0048518)

Take Fig. 6.1a as an example, the unlinked concepts *"siderophore metabolic process"* (GO:0009237) and *"peptide metabolic process"* (GO:0006518) differ in the first word and derive an unlinked ITP ([*siderophore*], [*peptide*]). In Fig. 6.2b, the linked concepts *"regulation of synaptic metaplasticity"* (GO:0031916) and *"regulation of biological process"* (GO:0050789) differ in the third and fourth words and derive a linked ITP ([*synaptic, metaplasticity*], [*biological, process*]).

Detection of Potential Inconsistencies

If the unlinked ITP derived from an unlinked PMCP and the linked ITP derived from a linked PMCP are the same, we consider the two PMCPs as a potential subtype inconsistency. For instance, the unlinked PMCP (GO:0009237, GO:0006518) in Fig. 6.1a and the linked PMCP (GO:0019290, GO:0043043) in Fig. 6.1b is considered a potential subtype inconsistency, since they derive the same ITP ([*siderophore*], [*peptide*]).

The unlinked PMCP (GO:0031918, GO:0048518) in Fig. 6.2a and the linked PMCP (GO:0031916, GO:0050789) in Fig. 6.2b are considered as a potential subtype inconsistency, since they derive the same ITP ([*synaptic, metaplasticity*], [*biological, process*]). Similarly, Figs. 6.3 and 6.4 give examples of potential subtype inconsistencies in NCIt and SNOMED CT, respectively.

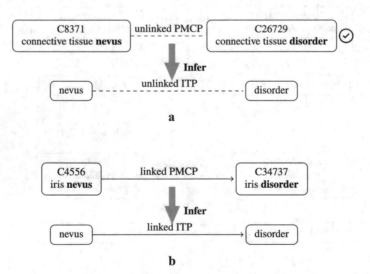

Fig. 6.3 a: An unlinked PMCP with diff 3 in NCIt and its unlinked ITP derived; **b**: A linked PMCP with diff 3 in NCIt and its linked ITP derived. This example reveals a potentially **missing subtype relation** in **a**, that is, *"connective tissue nevus"* (C8371) *is-a* *"connective tissue disorder"* (C26729)

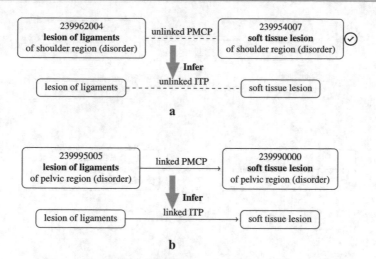

Fig. 6.4 **a**: An unlinked PMCP with diff 3 in SNOMED CT and its unlinked ITP derived; **b**: A linked PMCP with diff 3 in SNOMED CT and its linked ITP derived. This example reveals a potentially **missing subtype relation** in **a**, that is, "*lesion of ligaments of shoulder region (disorder)*" (239962004) *is-a* "*soft tissue lesion of shoulder region (disorder)*" (239954007)

Evaluation of Detected Potential Inconsistencies

Evaluation by Domain Experts A random sample of potential subtype inconsistencies detected in GO was selected and evaluated by two domain experts (authors EWH and HNBM), to evaluate the effectiveness of our approach in detecting inconsistencies. The two domain experts reviewed and discussed the samples together.

We classify the detected potential inconsistencies into three categories during the evaluation: missing subtype relations, incorrect existing subtype relations, and false positives. Given an inconsistency I consisting of an unlinked PMCP (u_1, u_2) and a linked PMCP (l_1, l_2), we describe each of the three categories in detail as follows.

- Missing Subtype Relations: If the concepts in the unlinked PMCP (u_1, u_2) form a valid subtype relation, then it is regarded as a missing subtype (i.e., u_1 should be a subtype of u_2). For instance, in Fig. 6.2a, the concepts in the unlinked PMCP (GO:0031918, GO:0048518) indeed form a valid subtype relation; thus, there is a missing subtype relation—"*positive regulation of synaptic metaplasticity*" (GO:0031918) should be a subtype of "*positive regulation of biological process*" (GO:0048518).
- Incorrect Existing Subtype Relations: If the concepts in the linked PMCP (l_1, l_2) are found to be an invalid subtype relation, then it is regarded as an incorrect existing subtype relation (i.e., l_1 should not be a subtype of l_2). For example, in Fig. 6.1b, the concepts in the linked PMCP (GO:0019290, GO:0043043) are found to form an invalid subtype relation because the definition of siderophores clearly indicates that some are not peptides, for

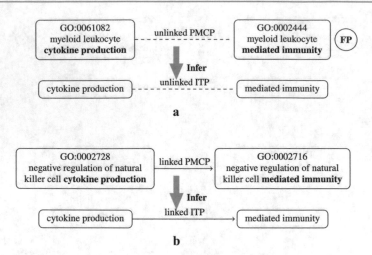

Fig. 6.5 a: An unlinked PMCP with diff 2 in GO and its unlinked ITP derived; **b**: A linked PMCP with diff 2 in GO and its linked ITP derived. Evaluated by the domain experts, the unlinked PMCP in **a** is an invalid subtype relation, the linked PMCP in **b** is a valid subtype relation, and therefore the potential inconsistency in this example is a **false positive** (**FP**)

example quinolbactin produced by Pseudomonas fluorescens [118]. That is, "*siderophore biosynthetic process*" (GO:0019290) should not be a subtype of "*peptide biosynthetic process*" (GO:0043043).

- False Positives: If the concepts in the linked PMCP (l_1, l_2) indeed form a valid subtype relation and the concepts in the unlinked PMCP (u_1, u_2) are found to be an invalid subtype relation, then I is regarded as a false positive. For example, the concepts in the linked PMCP (GO:0002728, GO:0002716) in Fig. 6.5b indeed forms a valid subtype relation, and the unlinked PMCP (GO:0061082, GO:0002444) in Fig. 6.5a does not form a valid subtype relation. Therefore, the inconsistency shown in Fig. 6.5 is a false positive.

Cross-terminology Evaluation based on UMLS We also leveraged external knowledge in UMLS (i.e., other terminologies in UMLS) to identify supporting evidence for detected potential subtype inconsistencies, which indicates the extent to which cross-terminology can help with validating whether a detected subtype inconsistency is a missing subtype relation. We performed such automated cross-terminology evaluation for GO, NCIt, and SNOMED CT, respectively.

Given a terminology, we perform a systematic check for each detected potential subtype inconsistency I. Assume that (u_1, u_2) is the unlinked PMCP involved in the inconsistency I. Then we map concepts u_1 and u_2 to the corresponding UMLS concepts m_1 and m_2. If there exists a path p from m_1 to m_2 in UMLS such that $p = m_1, m_{i_1}, m_{i_2}, \ldots, m_{i_k}, m_2$ where m_1 is-a m_{i_1}, m_{i_1} is-a m_{i_2}, ..., and m_{i_k} is-a m_2, then we say that there is evidence in UMLS supporting that u_1 is a subtype of u_2. Note that the subtype relations along the path may be from different terminologies. For instance, in Fig. 6.3, the path from "*connective tissues nevus*" (C8371) to "*connective tissue disorder*" (C26729) in UMLS was found through terminologies SNOMED CT and MEDCIN.

6.1.2   Overall Results, Domain Expert and Cross-Terminology Evaluation

A total of 4,841 potential inconsistencies were found in the 03/28/2017 release of GO, 2,677 in the 07/2018 release of NCIt, and 53,782 in the 01/03/2018 release of SNOMED CT US edition, respectively.

A random sample of 211 detected inconsistencies was reviewed by the domain experts, and 124 were found to be valid. Among the valid inconsistencies, 94 were missing subtype relations and 30 were incorrect existing subtype relations. The overall precision of the method is 58.77% (124/211).

The UMLS-based evaluation identified supporting evidence for missing subtype relations involved in 26 detected inconsistencies in GO, 306 in NCIt, and 1,940 in SNOMED CT, respectively. For detailed results, please see [119, 120].

6.1.3   Further Discussion About the Results and the Approach

Analysis of Failure Cases

The invalid inconsistencies confirmed by the domain experts are considered false positives. Figure 6.5 shows an example of false positives, where the linked PMCP is correct, and the unlinked PMCP is incorrect. This is due to the existing relation in GO in Fig. 6.5b being a regulation of a complex pathway of two concepts that could be hierarchically related while the suggested relation in Fig. 6.5a being the concepts themselves which cannot be related. In scenarios such as these, the suitable relationship is *part-of* instead of *is-a*. An analogy could be made to the two concepts *Engine* and *Cylinder block*. The regulation of the *Cylinder block* may be a subclass of regulation of the *Engine*, but inferring *Cylinder block is-a Engine* is incorrect. However, it is correct that *Cylinder block* is *part_of Engine*.

Another scenario of false positives is that the ITPs involve general terms such as (*senescence, development*), which may not be suitable to serve as a good candidate to detect subtype inconsistencies. An example of unlinked PMCPs is "*floral organ senescence*" (GO:0080187) and "*floral organ development*" (GO:0048437). Senescence is not a specific type of development, rather it is a state within the process of development and would more accurately be considered a component of development. Therefore, there should be a *part-of* relation between "*floral organ senescence*" (GO:0080187) and "*floral organ development*" (GO:0048437), which is already existent in the current GO.

Limitations and Future Work

In this approach, we limited the definition of PMCPs to concept-pairs having the same number of words. However, it should be noted that ITPs could be derived by any pair of concepts without such a restriction. We plan to perform such an analysis to study whether disregarding the restriction will affect the overall performance of our approach.

Another limitation of this approach is that we did not take into account the granularity of the inferred term pairs when generating potential inconsistencies. It would be useful to leverage some weight functions to inferred term pairs so that more general terms are given a less weight and more specific terms are given a higher weight when generating potential inconsistencies.

Additionally, we only performed automated evaluation by leveraging external knowledge in UMLS which showed limited supporting evidence: 0.54% (=26/4841) for GO, 11.43% (=306/2677) for NCIt, and 3.61% (=1940/53782) for SNOMED CT. It would be interesting to further investigate methods to leverage other external knowledge such as biomedical literature to automatically identify supporting evidence for detected potential inconsistencies and reduce domain experts' manual effort.

Conclusion: The focus of this section was on a lexical-based inference approach to audit biomedical terminologies based on the inconsistencies of inferred term-pairs derived from linked and unlinked concept-pairs. We applied this approach to GO, NCIt, and SNOMED CT respectively to detect potential subtype inconsistencies. Domain experts perform an evaluation on a random sample of inconsistencies in GO that revealed our approach achieved a precision of 58.77%. We also performed a preliminary study on a UMLS-based method to automatically identify supporting evidence of missing subtype relations to understand to what extent the external knowledge in UMLS can help with reducing the manual evaluation effort required from domain experts. The results demonstrated that the lexical-based inference approach is a promising method to detect potential subtype inconsistencies, which indicate missing subtype relations as well as incorrect subtype relations. This approach is also applicable to other biomedical terminologies for quality assurance analysis.

6.2   Subsumption-Based Sub-Term Inference

In this section, we introduce a novel Subsumption-based Sub-term Inference Framework (SSIF) for uncovering not only missing relations but also erroneous relations in the Gene Ontology (GO). SSIF will leverage a sequence-based term-algebra to analyze sophisticated lexical features of GO concepts and pinpoint the exact locations of quality issues.

6.2.1   Components of SSIF

SSIF is developed by leveraging both the underlying hierarchical structure of GO and a novel term-algebra. SSIF contains three main components: (1) a sequence-based representation of GO concepts constructed using part-of-speech (POS) tagging, sub-concept matching, and antonym tagging; (2) a formulation of algebraic operations for the development of a term-algebra based on the sequence-based representation, that leverages subsumption-based longest subsequence alignment; and (3) the construction of a set of conditional rules for backward subsumption inference aimed at uncovering problematic *is-a* relations in GO.

We first parse the OWL file of the 2018-10-03 release of GO to extract all the concepts and *is-a* relations in GO. Then we compute the *is-a* transitive closure to get all the direct and indirect *is-a* relations.

Sequence-Based Representation of GO Concepts

It has been pointed out that over 65% of GO concepts (or terms) contain another GO term as a proper substring [121]. For instance, *"negative regulation of cellular protein catabolic process"* (GO:1903363) contains the term *"regulation of cellular protein catabolic process"* (GO:1903362) as a proper substring. We refer to the proper substring as a sub-concept of the original concept. In addition, we consider those GO concepts containing only alphanumeric characters, constituting almost 90% of GO concepts.

We represent each GO concept with a sequence of primitive elements, where a primitive element can be a single word or a sub-concept. Given an input concept C, we denote its sequence of elements $E(C)$ as $[e_1, e_2, e_3, \ldots, e_n]$. We further annotate the elements with tags and form the corresponding sequence of tags $T(C)$, denoted as $[t_1, t_2, t_3, \ldots, t_n]$ where tag t_i corresponds to element e_i. The following three tagging processes are performed: POS tagging, sub-concept tagging, and antonym tagging.

POS Tagging We leverage the Stanford Parser [122] to parse and annotate the GO terms to obtain sequence-based representations with tagged annotations for concepts. For example, the concept $C =$ *"negative regulation of cellular protein catabolic process"* (GO:1903363) is represented and annotated as follows:

   $E(C) =$ [*negative, regulation, of, cellular, protein, catabolic, process*],
   $T(C) =$ [*JJ, NN, IN, JJ, NN, JJ, NN*],
where *JJ, NN,* and *IN* are the POS tags denoting adjective, noun, and preposition or subordinating conjunction, respectively.

Sub-concept Tagging After the POS tagging, we further detect sub-concepts contained in the concepts. Then we replace the substrings corresponding to the subconcepts with their GO identifiers. More specifically, for a concept C with sequence-based representation $E(C) = [e_1, e_2, e_3, \ldots, e_n]$ and annotation $T(C) = [t_1, t_2, t_3, \ldots, t_n]$, if substring $[e_j, e_{j+1}, \ldots e_k]$ $(1 \le j \le k \le n)$ is also a GO concept S whose identifier is $I(S)$, then we

Table 6.1 Sequence representations for concept $C =$ "*negative regulation of cellular protein catabolic process*" (GO:1903363)

Sequence representation—$E(C)$	Tag annotation—$T(C)$
negative, GO:1903362	*JJ, SC*
negative, regulation, of, GO:0044257	*JJ, NN, IN, SC*
negative, regulation, of, cellular, GO:0030163	*JJ, NN, IN, JJ, SC*
negative, regulation, of, cellular, protein, GO:0009056	*JJ, NN, IN, JJ, NN, SC*

update the representation as $E(C) = [e_1, e_2, \ldots, e_{j-1}, I(S), e_{k+1}, \ldots, e_n]$ and the annotation as $T(C) = [t_1, t_2, \ldots, t_{j-1}, SC, t_{k+1}, \ldots, t_n]$, where SC denotes the sub-concept tag.

For example, for the input concept $C =$ "*negative regulation of cellular protein catabolic process*" (GO:1903363), there are four sub-concepts detected: "*regulation of cellular protein catabolic process)*" (GO:1903362, "*cellular protein catabolic process*" (GO:0044257), "*protein catabolic process*" (GO:0030163), and "*catabolic process*" (GO:0009056). Note that these sub-concepts are overlapping with each other (i.e., sharing at least one word in common), in which cases we generate multiple representations for the input concept to handle the overlap. Therefore, the input concept C has four different representations (see Table 6.1) corresponding to the four sub-concepts detected.

Table 6.2 shows the sequence-based representations and tag annotations for the concept $C =$ "*innate immune response activating cell surface receptor signaling pathway*" (GO:0002220), which contains the following sub-concepts: "*innate immune response*" (GO:0045087), "*immune response*" (GO: 0006955), "*cell*" (GO:0005623), "*cell surface*" (GO:0009986), "*signaling*" (GO:0023052), and "*cell surface receptor signaling pathway*" (GO:0007166). A total of six representations are generated to capture the overlaps among sub-concepts (see Table 6.2).

Antonym Tagging To annotate concepts involving words with antonyms, we leverage a comprehensive collection of antonym pairs provided by WordNet (https://wordnet.princeton. edu/), the most well-known lexical database for English. If there exists an element e_i of $E(C)$ belonging to the antonym collection, then we annotate e_i with the *ANT* tag in addition to its original tag. For instance, for the concept $C =$ "*negative regulation of cellular protein catabolic process*" (GO:1903363) (in Table 6.1), its first element *negative* involves the antonym pair (*positive, negative*), thus we add the *ANT* tag for *negative* (as shown in Table 6.3). Note that the *ANT* does not replace the original POS tag but rather serves as an additional tag for the element, indicating that the element *negative* is an adjective and has an antonym. We denote the antonym of element e_i as $\neg e_i$.

Table 6.2 Sequence representations for concept $C = innate\ immune\ response\ activating\ cell\ surface$ *receptor signaling pathway (GO:0002220)*

Sequence representation—$E(C)$
Tag annotation—$T(C)$
GO:0045087, activating, GO:0005623, surface, receptor, GO:0023052, pathway
SC, VBG, SC, NN, NN, SC, NN
GO:0045087, activating, GO:0009986, receptor, GO:0023052, pathway
SC, VBG, SC, NN, SC, NN
GO:0045087, activating, GO:0007166
SC, VBG, SC
innate, GO:0006955, activating, GO:0005623, surface, receptor, GO:0023052, pathway
JJ, SC, VBG, SC, NN, NN, SC, NN
innate, GO:0006955, activating, GO:0009986, receptor, GO:0023052, pathway
JJ, SC, VBG, SC, NN, SC, NN
innate, GO:0006955, activating, GO:0007166
JJ, SC, VBG, SC

Table 6.3 Sequence representations for concept $C = $ *"negative regulation of cellular protein catabolic process"* (GO:1903363) after antonym tagging

Sequence representation—$E(C)$	Tag annotation—$T(C)$
negative, GO:1903362	JJ/ANT, SC
negative, regulation, of, GO:0044257	JJ/ANT, NN, IN, SC
negative, regulation, of, cellular, GO:0030163	JJ/ANT, NN, IN, JJ, SC
negative, regulation, of, cellular, protein, GO:0009056	JJ/ANT, NN, IN, JJ, NN, SC

Algebraic Operations

Given two sequences of elements X and Y, if the term corresponding to X is a GO concept and a subtype (direct or indirect) of the term corresponding to Y, we say that X and Y have a subsumption relation, denoted as $X \preceq Y$; otherwise, we say that X and Y do not have a subsumption relation, denoted as $X \not\preceq Y$. In particular, we assume $X \preceq X$ for any sequence of elements X.

Next we define the subsumption-based longest common subsequence between two sequences of elements $X = [x_1, x_2, \ldots, x_m]$ and $Y = [y_1, y_2, \ldots, y_n]$. Let $X_i = [x_1, x_2, \ldots, x_i]$ and $Y_j = [y_1, y_2, \ldots, y_j]$ be the length i prefixes of X and length j prefixes of Y respectively, then the subsumption-based longest common subsequence between X_i and Y_j, $SLCS(X_i, Y_j)$, is defined as follows:

$$SLCS(X_i, Y_j) = \begin{cases} \emptyset & \text{if } i = 0 \text{ or } j = 0 \\ [SLCS(X_{i-1}, Y_{j-1}), x_i] & \text{if } i, j > 0 \text{ and } x_i \preceq y_j \\ [SLCS(X_{i-1}, Y_{j-1}), y_j] & \text{if } i, j > 0 \text{ and } y_j \preceq x_i \\ [longest(SLCS(X_i, Y_{j-1}), SLCS(X_{i-1}, Y_j))] & \text{if } i, j > 0 \text{ and } x_i \npreceq y_j \text{ and } y_j \npreceq x_i. \end{cases}$$

Hence, the subsumption-based longest common subsequence between X and Y, $SLCS$ $(X, Y) = SLCS(X_m, Y_n)$. For instance, consider the two concepts $C_1 = $ "*negative regulation by host of symbiont molecular function*" (GO: 0052405) and $C_2 = $ "*positive regulation by host of symbiont catalytic activity*" (GO:0043947), as well as their sequence representations [*negative, regulation, by, host, of, symbiont, GO:0003674*] and [*positive, regulation, by, host, of, symbiont, GO:0003824*]. Since "*catalytic activity*" (GO:0003824) is a subtype of "*molecular function*" (GO:0003674), we have $SLCS(C_1, C_2) = $ [*regulation, by, host, of, symbiont, GO:0003824*].

The subsumption-based longest common subsequence between sequences of elements allows us to define an algebraic operation *intersection* ($\sqcap$) as follows. Given two sequences of elements X and Y, there are two possible cases:

- Case I: $X \preceq Y$

  In this case, we define $X \sqcap Y = X$. That is to say, if the term corresponding to X is a subtype of (or more specific than) the term corresponding to Y, then $X \sqcap Y$ is defined as the sequence of the more specific term. For example, since *catabolic process (GO:0009056)* $\preceq$ *metabolic process (GO:0008152)*, we have *catabolic process (GO:0009056)* $\sqcap$ *metabolic process (GO:0008152)* = *catabolic process (GO:0009056)*. In particular, we define $X \sqcap X = X$ for any sequence of elements X. For instance, *protein* $\sqcap$ *protein* = *protein*.

- Case II: $X \npreceq Y$

  Suppose the subsumption-based longest common subsequence between two concepts $X = [x_1, x_2, \ldots, x_m]$ and $Y = [y_1, y_2, \ldots, y_n]$ is $SLCS(X, Y) = [e_1, e_2, \ldots, e_s]$, where $s \leq m$ and $s \leq n$. Then we define $X \sqcap Y$ as follows:

  1. If $s = m = n$, then $X \sqcap Y$ is defined as the sequence obtained by performing intersections between elements in X and Y, i.e.,

$$X \sqcap Y = [(x_1 \sqcap y_1), (x_2 \sqcap y_2), \ldots, (x_s \sqcap y_s)]$$
$$= [e_1, e_2, \ldots, e_s] = SLCS(X, Y).$$

For instance, for $X = $ [*cytoplasmic microtubule (GO:0005881), depolymerization*] and $Y = $ [*astral microtubule (GO:0000235), depolymerization*], since *astral microtubule (GO:0000235)* $\preceq$ *cytoplasmic microtubule (GO:0005881)*, we have

$$X \sqcap Y = [(cytoplasmic\ microtubule\ (GO{:}0005881)\ \sqcap$$
$$astral\ microtubule\ (GO{:}0000235)),$$
$$(depolymerization\ \sqcap\ depolymerization)]$$
$$= [astral\ microtubule\ (GO{:}0000235),\ depolymerization]$$
$$= Y.$$

2. If $s = m$ and $s < n$, then $X \sqcap Y$ is defined as the sequence obtained by replacing elements in Y with the corresponding elements in $SLCS(X, Y)$, that is, performing intersections between elements in X and Y corresponding to those in $SLCS(X, Y)$ while keeping the remaining elements in Y intact. Take $X = [protein,\ catabolic\ process\ (GO{:}0009056)]$ and $Y = [cellular,\ protein,\ metabolic\ process\ (GO{:}0008152)]$ as an example, since $catabolic\ process\ (GO{:}0009056) \preceq metabolic\ process\ (GO{:}0008152)$, we have $SLCS(X, Y) = [protein,\ catabolic\ process\ (GO{:}0009056)]$ and

$$X \sqcap Y = [cellular,\ (protein\ \sqcap\ protein),$$
$$(catabolic\ process\ (GO{:}0009056)\ \sqcap$$
$$metabolic\ process\ (GO{:}0008152))]$$
$$= [cellular,\ protein,\ catabolic\ process\ (GO{:}0009056)]$$

3. Similarly, if $s < m$ and $s = n$, then we define $X \sqcap Y$ as the sequence obtained by replacing elements in X with the corresponding elements in $SLCS(X, Y)$, that is, performing intersections between elements in X and Y corresponding to those in $SLCS(X, Y)$ while keeping the remaining elements in X intact.
4. In all other cases, $X \sqcap Y$ is defined as $\emptyset$.

Conditional Rules for Backward Subsumption-Based Inference

Based on the above-defined algebraic operations, we introduce three conditional rules for performing backward subsumption-based inference in order to identify potential problematic *is-a* relations in GO: missing *is-a* relations or erroneous *is-a* relations.

Monotonicity Rule Given two GO concepts A and B such that $E(A)$ and $E(B)$ have the same number of elements, $E(A) = [a_1, a_2, a_3, \ldots, a_n]$ and $E(B) = [b_1, b_2, b_3, \ldots, b_n]$. A suggestion of $A \preceq B$ or A *is-a* B (a potentially missing *is-a* relation) may be made, if the following conditions are met:

1. $a_i \preceq b_i$ holds for all i ($1 \leq i \leq n$);
2. A is currently not a subtype of B; and
3. there does not exist an element a_i in $E(A)$ with a tag *ANT* such that $\neg a_i$ is in $E(B)$.

Fig. 6.6 An example of two
GO concepts satisfying the
monotonicity rule and
revealing a missing *is-a*
relation: *GO:0071450 is-a
GO:0071241* (see the bolded,
dashed arrow)

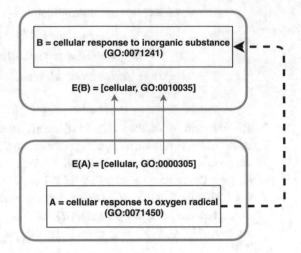

Take two concepts $A =$ "*cellular response to oxygen radical*" (GO:0071450) and $B =$
"*cellular response to inorganic substance*" (GO:0071241) shown in Fig. 6.6 as an example, where the sequence-based representations of A and B are $E(A) = [cellular, response$
to oxygen radical (GO:0000305)] and $E(B) = [cellular, response to inorganic substance$
(GO:0010035)], respectively. Since *cellular* $\preceq$ *cellular* and *response to oxygen radical
(GO:0000305)* $\preceq$ *response to inorganic substance (GO:0010035)*, a suggestion of $A \preceq B$
may be made, that is, "*cellular response to oxygen radical*" (GO:0071450) is a subtype of
"*cellular response to inorganic substance*" (GO:0071241).

Note that the validity of the suggested missing *is-a* relation still need to be verified by
domain experts. If the suggested missing *is-a* relation is valid, then it is indeed a missing
is-a relation (e.g., Fig. 6.6). If the suggested missing *is-a* relation is invalid, but there exists j
($1 \leq j \leq n$) such that $a_j \preceq b_j$ is an erroneous relation which leads to the invalid suggestion,
then $a_j \preceq b_j$ can be identified as an erroneous relation in GO.

For example, in Fig. 6.7, concept $A =$ "*pyridine nucleotide catabolic process*"
(GO:0019364) has a sequence-based representation $E(A) = [pyridine, nucleotide catabolic$
process (GO:0009166)] and concept $B =$ "*pyridine biosynthetic process*" (GO:0019364) has
a sequence-based representation $E(B) = [pyridine, biosynthetic process (GO:0009058)]$.
Since *pyridine* $\preceq$ *pyridine* and *GO:0009166* $\preceq$ *GO:0009058*, a suggestion of "*pyridine nucleotide catabolic process*" (GO:0019364) *is-a* "*pyridine biosynthetic process*"
(GO:0046220) may be made. However, this is an invalid suggestion due to an erroneous
existing *is-a* relation: *nucleotide catabolic process (GO:0009166)* $\preceq$ *biosynthetic process
(GO:0009058)*, since catabolism is not anabolism (biosynthesis).

Intersection Rule Suppose A, B, and C are GO concepts such that $A \preceq B$ and $A \preceq C$. A
suggestion of $A \preceq B \sqcap C$ (a potentially missing *is-a* relation) may be made, if the following
conditions are satisfied:

Fig. 6.7 An example of two GO concepts satisfying the monotonicity rule and revealing an erroneous *is-a* relation: "*nucleotide catabolic process*" (GO:0009166) *is-a* "*biosynthetic process*" (GO:0009058) (see the bolded arrow with a cross)

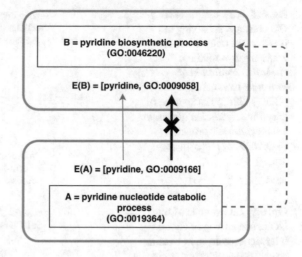

1. $B \sqcap C$ is also a GO concept;
2. $B \sqcap C \preceq B$ and $B \sqcap C \preceq C$;
3. A is currently not a subtype of $B \sqcap C$; and
4. there does not exist an element a_i in $E(A)$ with a tag *ANT* such that $\neg a_i$ is in $E(B)$.

Intuitively, it is suggested that $B \sqcap C$ is the maximal concept that is more specific than both B and C.

For instance, in Fig. 6.8, concept $A =$ "*negative regulation of ornithine catabolic process*" (GO:1903267) is a subtype of concept $B =$ "*negative regulation of cellular amine metabolic process*" (GO:0033239) and also a subtype of concept $C =$ "*regulation of cellular catabolic process*" (GO:0031329). $B \sqcap C =$ "*negative regulation of cellular amine catabolic process*" (GO:0033242) is also a GO concept, which is a subtype of A and B as well. Therefore a suggestion of A *is-a* $B \sqcap C$ may be made, that is, "*negative regulation of ornithine catabolic process*" (GO:1903267) is a subtype of "*negative regulation of cellular amine catabolic process*" (GO:0033242).

If the suggested missing *is-a* relation is valid, then it is indeed a missing *is-a* relation (e.g., Fig. 6.8). If the suggested missing *is-a* relation is invalid, but there exists erroneous *is-a* relation(s) among $A \preceq B$, $A \preceq C$, $B \sqcap C \preceq B$ and $B \sqcap C \preceq C$ leading to the invalid suggestion, then erroneous *is-a* relation(s) in GO can be identified.

For example, in Fig. 6.9, concept $A =$ "*positive regulation of B cell deletion*" (GO:0002869) is a subtype of concept $B =$ "*regulation of acute inflammatory response*" (GO:0002673) and also a subtype of concept $C =$ "*positive regulation of biological process*" (GO:0048518). $B \sqcap C =$ "*positive regulation of acute inflammatory response*" (GO:0002675) is also a GO concept, which is a subtype of A and B as well. Therefore a suggestion of A *is-a* $B \sqcap C$ may be made, that is, "*positive regulation of B cell deletion*" (GO:0002869) is a subtype of "*positive regulation of acute inflammatory response*" (GO:0002675). However, this is an invalid suggestion due to an erroneous existing *is-a*

Fig. 6.8 An example of four GO concepts satisfying the intersection rule and revealing a missing *is-a* relation: *"negative regulation of ornithine catabolic process"* (GO:1903267) is a subtype of *"negative regulation of cellular amine catabolic process"* (GO:0033242) (see the red arrow)

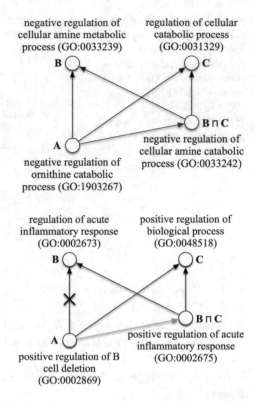

negative regulation of cellular amine metabolic process (GO:0033239)

regulation of cellular catabolic process (GO:0031329)

B ⊓ C
negative regulation of cellular amine catabolic process (GO:0033242)

negative regulation of ornithine catabolic process (GO:1903267)

Fig. 6.9 An example of four GO concepts satisfying the intersection rule and revealing an erroneous existing relation: *"positive regulation of B cell deletion"* (GO:0002869) *is-a* *"regulation of acute inflammatory response"* (GO:0002673) (see the red arrow with a cross)

regulation of acute inflammatory response (GO:0002673)

positive regulation of biological process (GO:0048518)

B ⊓ C
positive regulation of acute inflammatory response (GO:0002675)

positive regulation of B cell deletion (GO:0002869)

relation: *"positive regulation of B cell deletion"* (GO:0002869) *is-a* *"regulation of acute inflammatory response"* (GO:0002673). The main purpose of B cell deletion is to produce immune tolerance. Since tolerance induction is a long process (not something that is acute), it is incorrect that *"positive regulation of B cell deletion"* (GO:0002869) is a subtype of *"regulation of acute inflammatory response"* (GO:0002673).

Sub-concept Rule Given a concept C with a sequence-based representation as $E(C) = [e_1, e_2, e_3, \ldots, e_{n-1}, e_n]$ and a tag annotation as $T(C) = [t_1, t_2, t_3, \ldots, t_{n-1}, t_n]$. A suggestion of $C \preceq e_n$ (a potentially missing *is-a* relation) may be made, if the following conditions are met:

1. $t_n = SC$, i.e., the last element e_n is also a GO concept;
2. $t_i \in \{NN, JJ, SC\}$ for each i ($1 \leq i \leq n-1$), i.e., the tags $t_1, t_2, t_3, \ldots, t_{n-1}$ are either noun, adjective, or sub-concept;
3. C is currently not a subtype of e_n; and
4. there does not exist an element a_i in $E(C)$ with a tag ANT such that $\neg a_i$ is in e_n.

For instance, concept $C = $ *"nerve growth factor receptor binding"* (GO:0005163) has a sequence-based representation $E(C) = [$*nerve, growth factor receptor binding*

(GO:0070851)] with a tag annotation $T(C) = [NN, SC]$. Since the last element *growth factor receptor binding (GO:0070851)* is also a GO concept and the remaining element *nerve* is a noun, a suggestion of "*nerve growth factor receptor binding*" (GO:0005163) *is-a* "*growth factor receptor binding*" (GO:0070851) may be made.

If the suggested missing *is-a* relation is valid, then it is indeed a missing *is-a* relation. Note that the sub-concept rule does not leverage any existing *is-a* relation to make suggestions, thus it can not reveal erroneous existing *is-a* relations in GO.

Evaluation

A random sample of potentially missing *is-a* relations is selected and evaluated by two domain experts. The evaluation is performed independently by each domain expert and the disagreements between the two experts are resolved by discussion. For the monotonicity rule and intersection rule, domain experts are also provided with the existing *is-a* relations in GO that are leveraged to suggest the potentially missing *is-a* relations.

The validity of each suggested missing *is-a* relation in the random sample is evaluated by the domain experts. If the suggested missing *is-a* relation is valid, then it is indeed a missing *is-a* relation and considered as a true positive; if the suggested missing *is-a* relation is invalid due to existing erroneous relation(s), then the erroneous *is-a* relation(s) are identified as valid and considered as true positive(s); and all the other cases are considered as false positives. The precision of SSIF according to each rule can be calculated by dividing the number of true positives by the total number of true positives and false positives.

6.2.2   Overall Results and Evaluation

We briefly discuss our findings as follows. For further details about the results, please see [123].

Summary Results

For the 2018-10-03 release of GO, a total of 40,030 (out of 44,942) concepts were annotated with sequence-based representation. Among these, 30,086 concepts involve sub-concepts and 13,163 involve antonyms. Monotonicity, Intersection, and Sub-concept rules suggested 819, 691, and 669 rules respectively. In total, three conditional rules suggested 1,938 unique potentially missing *is-a* relations. The monotonicity and intersection rules leveraged 2,436 existing *is-a* relations to make these suggestions. Note that certain potentially missing *is-a* relations can be obtained by multiple rules. For instance, 11 potentially missing *is-a* relations can be obtained by both the sub-concept rule and monotonicity rule; 228 can be obtained by the monotonicity rule and intersection rule; and 1 can be obtained by all the three conditional rules.

Evaluation Results

A total of 210 potentially missing *is-a* relations were randomly selected and evaluated by domain experts. There were 99 samples obtained from the Monotonicity rule of which 54 were found to be missing *is-a* relations and 6 were erroneous *is-a* relations (precision of 60.61%). Intersection rule obtained 81 samples in the evaluation sample of which 44 were missing *is-a* relations, and 5 were erroneous *is-a* relations (precision of 60.49%). Meanwhile, Sub-concept rule contained 63 samples of which 29 were deemed as missing *is-a* relations (precision of 46.03%).

6.2.3   Analysis of Results and Potential Directions

Analysis of False Positives

Although SSIF was capable of uncovering problematic *is-a* relations in GO, it cannot completely avoid false positives. For example, the sub-concept rule suggested "*nuclear membrane mitotic spindle pole body tethering complex*" (GO:0106084) is a subtype of "*tethering complex*" (GO:0099023). However, this relation is invalid, since "*tethering complex*" is defined as a complex that plays a role in vesicle tethering, while "*nuclear membrane mitotic spindle pole body tethering complex*" is tethering non-vesicle cellular components. Note that "*tethering complex*" has been renamed as "*vesicle tethering complex*" in the current release of GO, in which case SSIF will not make the invalid suggestion of *GO:0106084 is-a GO:0099023*.

The monotonicity rule suggested "*negative regulation of renal output by angiotensin*" (GO:0003083) *is-a* "*negative regulation of systemic arterial blood pressure*" (GO:0003085). This is an invalid *is-a* relation because "*negative regulation of renal output by angiotensin*" (GO:0003083) is actually a subtype of "*positive regulation of systemic arterial blood pressure*" (GO:0003084). Although this invalid *is-a* relation was obtained by an existing *is-a* relation: "*regulation of renal output by angiotensin*" (GO:0002019) is a subtype of "*regulation of systemic arterial blood pressure*" (GO:0003073), the latter relation is valid as the two concepts do not specify a qualifier of positive or negative.

The intersection rule suggested "*peptide cross-linking via an oxazole or thiazole*" (GO:0018157) *is-a* "*cellular macromolecule biosynthetic process*" (GO:0034645). This potentially missing *is-a* relation was obtained by two existing *is-a* relations: "*peptide cross-linking via an oxazole or thiazole*" (GO:0018157) *is-a* "*cellular macromolecule metabolic process*" (GO:0044260) and "*peptide cross-linking via an oxazole or thiazole*" (GO:0018157) *is-a* "*cellular biosynthetic process*" (GO:0044249). Since biosynthesis is for the oxazole or thiazole, but not for the macromolecule (which is simply being modified), the former relation is invalid while the latter two existing relations are valid.

As it was seen in the evaluation results, the precision of SSIF according to the sub-concept rule is lower than that of the monotonicity rule and intersection rule. Through manual review of the false positives obtained by the sub-concept rule, we found that there were 11 of the suggested potentially missing *is-a* relations which already have a *part-of* relation in GO. For instance, the sub-concept suggested "*basal plasma membrane*" (GO:0009925) *is-a* "*plasma membrane*" (GO:0005886). However the two concepts already have a *part-of* relation.

Limitations and Future Work

A limitation of this approach is that we only focused on suggesting problematic *is-a* relations in GO. As mentioned earlier, the sub-concept rule suggested some invalid *is-a* relations which already have a *part-of* relation. We plan to further investigate other types of problematic relations in GO including *part-of*. Regarding the identification of erroneous *is-a* relations in terms of the monotonicity rule and intersection rule, although SSIF requires significantly less manual effort from domain experts than most other ontology auditing approaches (by providing rationales for the suggestions of problematic *is-a* relations), domain experts still need to review the provided existing *is-a* relations that were leveraged to make the suggestion and determine if there is any erroneous relation(s) can be identified or the original suggestion is a false positive. It would be desirable to develop an automated approach that can directly detect erroneous *is-a* relations to further reduce domain experts' manual review effort.

Conclusion: In this section, we introduced SSIF, a subsumption-based sub-term inference framework, to identify problematic *is-a* relations in GO. SSIF models GO concepts in a sequence-based representation, formulates a term-algebra, and leverages three conditional rules to perform backward subsumption inference, in order to automatically suggest potentially missing *is-a* relations, which may further reveal erroneous *is-a* relations. Since SSIF leverages the hierarchical structure and the features of concept names, which are inherent and fundamental to biomedical terminologies, it is generally applicable to audit other biomedical terminologies.

6.3   Transformation-Based Method

In this section, we discuss a novel transformation-based auditing method that leverages the knowledge in the Unified Medical Language System (UMLS) to systematically identify missing hierarchical *is-a* relations in the source terminologies. Quality improvement of the source terminologies will in turn enhance the qualities of the UMLS knowledge sources.

This method takes full advantage of the rich knowledge provided by the UMLS for auditing and improving the qualities of its source terminologies, which in turn enhances the quality of the UMLS. Unlike the traditional terminology auditing methods that often rely on the knowledge within the terminology itself (i.e., internal knowledge), our method leverages not only the terminology itself but also the knowledge from other multiple terminologies in the UMLS (i.e., both internal and external knowledge). This will result in newly identified missing *is-a* relations that would not be uncovered by only looking into one or two individual terminologies. In addition, unlike previous related work on auditing the UMLS that mainly focused on auditing high level views (e.g., semantic types, concepts/CUIs, relations between concepts), this approach intends to audit the UMLS source terminologies in the atom level.

6.3.1   Steps of the Transformation-Based Method

This approach is applied to the UMLS 2019AB release. Our method consists of four main steps to identify potentially missing *is-a* relations for each concept name in the UMLS: (1) parse the concept name and identify noun chunks; (2) generate replacement candidates for noun chunks; (3) perform concept name transformation and construct new potential concept names; and (4) map newly constructed concept names to atoms and identify potentially missing *is-a* relations in the source terminologies.

Parsing Concept Names
We first convert each concept name to lowercase. We then use spaCy [114], an open-source library for advanced NLP, to perform dependency parsing and identify noun chunks within concept names. For example, Fig. 6.10 shows the dependency graph of the concept name *"Primary basal cell carcinoma of left eyelid"* where two base noun chunks can be identified: "primary basal cell carcinoma" and "left eyelid." Here a base noun chunk consists of a head (e.g., "carcinoma") plus words describing the head (e.g., "primary basal cell").[29] Note that "basal cell" is not a base noun chunk since it is used to modify or describe "carcinoma." Instead, we consider such noun phrases describing the head as secondary noun chunks. After the parsing, each concept name C can be represented as an ordered array of elements $[c_1, c_2, \ldots, c_n]$, where c_i can be a single word, a base noun chunk, or a secondary noun chunk. For instance, the concept name *"Primary basal cell carcinoma of left eyelid"* can be represented in two forms: (1) [primary basal cell carcinoma, of, left eyelid]; and (2) [primary, basal cell, carcinoma, of, left eyelid].

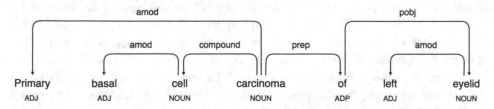

Fig. 6.10 Dependency graph of the concept name *"Primary basal cell carcinoma of left eyelid."*

Table 6.4 An example of the transformation process for *"Acute dacryoadenitis of left eye"*

Concept name	Acute dacryoadenitis of left eye
Representation ($[c_1, c_2, c_3]$)	[acute dacryoadenitis, of, left eye]
Replacement candidates for *"acute dacryoadenitis" (r1)*	{dacryoadenitis, inflammation of specific body systems, acute disease, acute inflammatory disease, inflammatory disorder, inflammatory disorder of head, disorder of eyelid or lacrimal system, disorder of lacrimal gland}
Replacement candidates for *"left eye" (r3)*	{organ of special sense, eye, subdivision of face}
Combinatorial replacements	[{acute dacryoadenitis, dacryoadenitis, inflammation of specific body systems, acute disease, acute inflammatory disease, inflammatory disorder, inflammatory disorder of head, disorder of eyelid or lacrimal system, disorder of lacrimal gland}, of, {left eye, organ of special sense, eye, subdivision of face}]
Potentially missing *is-a* relations detected in source terminologies	SNOMEDCT_US: *"acute dacryoadenitis of left eye"* is-a *"acute disease of eye"* MEDCIN: *"acute dacryoadenitis of left eye"* is-a *"inflammatory disorder of eye"*

Identifying Replacement Candidates

In this step, we identify replacement candidates that are more general than the noun chunks (base and secondary) in each concept name. If a noun chunk can be mapped to a UMLS atom (i.e., the noun chunk is also a concept name in an existing source terminology), then we consider the concept names of this atom's ancestors in its source terminology as replacement candidates for the noun chunk; otherwise, the noun chunk is considered as not having any replacement candidates. To avoid replacement candidates being too general, we leveraged ancestors of the atom within a distance of two levels using Depth-limited-search [124].

Take the concept name *"Acute dacryoadenitis of left eye"* in Table 6.4 as an example, it can be represented as an array [acute dacryoadenitis, of, left eye]. The noun chunk "acute dacryoadenitis" can be mapped to 9 atoms. For example, *A2889158* is an atom sourced from the SNOMED CT (US edition) with seven level-2 ancestors. After going through all the 9 atoms, the following replacement candidates for "acute dacryoadenitis" can be obtained: "disorder of lacrimal gland," "disorder of eyelid or lacrimal system," "dacryoadenitis," "inflammation of specific body systems," "acute inflammatory disease," "inflammatory disorder of head," "acute disease," and "inflammatory disorder."

Concept Name Transformation

For each concept name with noun chunk(s) such that the replacement candidates have been identified already, we replace the original noun chunk(s) with their corresponding candidates to generate new potential concept names, which may serve as supertypes of the original concept name (since the replacement candidates are more general than the original noun chunk). Formally, given a concept name C represented by $[c_1, c_2, \ldots, c_n]$ where there exists an i such that c_i is a base or secondary noun chunk and r_i is a set of replacement candidates for c_i, then we replace c_i with any candidate in r_i and concatenate the array as a string to construct new concept names that may serve as C's supertypes. If there are multiple such i's, we will perform combinatorial replacements for multiple i's.

Take the concept name "*Acute dacryoadenitis of left eye*" in Table 6.4 as an example. There are three elements in its array representation $[c_1, c_2, c_3]$ where c_1 and c_3 are base noun chunks. There are 8 replacement candidates for c_1 and 3 for c_3. A total of 35 new potential concept names can be obtained after the combinatory replacements for c_1 and c_3, including "*acute disease of eye*" and "*acute inflammatory disease of left eye*."

Identify Missing is-a Relations in Source Terminologies

In this step, we check if the newly generated concept names exist in the UMLS (i.e., exactly match the names of UMLS atoms) to identify potentially missing *is-a* relations between atoms in source terminologies. Given a concept name C (mapped to an atom AUI_C) and a potential concept name S serving as its supertype, if the following conditions hold:

1. S can be mapped to a UMLS atom AUI_S;
2. AUI_S comes from the same source terminology T as AUI_C;
3. currently, there is no *is-a* relation (either direct or indirect) between AUI_S and AUI_C claimed in T; and
4. AUI_C has the same semantic type as AUI_S, or the set of semantic types of AUI_C contains that of AUI_S as a subset,

then we consider there is a potentially missing *is-a* relation between AUI_C and AUI_S (i.e., AUI_C *is-a* AUI_S) in the terminology T. Note that missing *is-a* relations between atoms from different source terminologies are beyond the scope of this approach. The semantic type requirement of C and S is to avoid ambiguities caused by concept names which may have multiple meanings. For example, the concept name "*cold*" could refer to lower temperature (with a semantic type "*Natural Phenomenon or Process*") or a kind of disease (with a semantic type "*Disease or Syndrome*").

For "*acute dacryoadenitis of left eye*" in Table 6.4, after the transformation, "*acute disease of eye*" is one of its potential new concept names which can be mapped to atoms, while "*acute inflammatory disease of left eye*" cannot. By further mapping concept names to atoms, a potentially missing *is-a* relation between "*acute dacryoadenitis of left eye*" with AUI *A27761536* and "*acute disease of eye*" with AUI *A3463187* can be identified in the SNOMED CT.

It is worth noting that the potentially missing *is-a* relations identified by our method may contain redundancy. Here a missing *is-a* relation (say "*x is-a y*") identified in a terminology T is considered redundant, if there exists another missing *is-a* relation "*x is-a z*" identified in T such that y is currently an ancestor of z in T. In this case, if "*x is-a z*" is a valid missing *is-a* relation, then "*x is-a y*" can be implied as valid by "*x is-a z*" and "*z is-a y.*" Therefore, we further remove the potentially missing *is-a* relations that are redundant from the result.

6.3.2 Missing *is-a* Relations Identified, Evaluation, and Further Analysis

In the following subsections, we summarize the findings of this approach. For detailed results and analysis, please see [125].

Identifying Missing is-a Relations

We applied this method to the English-language concept names in the UMLS (2019AB release). In total, our method identified 42,362 potentially missing *is-a* relations from 13 source terminologies in the UMLS. 39,359 out of 42,362 are non-redundant.

Evaluation

To assess the effectiveness of our method for identifying missing *is-a* relations in the UMLS source terminologies, a sample of 200 *is-a* relations from SNOMED CT (the "*Clinical Finding*" subhierarchy) and a sample of 100 from the Gene Ontology were randomly selected. The samples were reviewed by domain experts. Domain experts verified that 173 out of 200 potentially missing *is-a* relations in the SNOMED CT (a precision of 86.5%) and 63 out of 100 in the Gene Ontology (a precision of 63%) are valid.

Analyses of False Positive Cases

Analyzing the evaluation results of the domain experts, it was noted that the main cause of false positives is that the biomedical meanings of replacement candidates are not considered to be more general than their corresponding noun chunks. This could relate to either incorrect existing *is-a* relations or different views of different terminologies. Take "*cellular response to beta-carotene*" *is-a* "*cellular response to vitamin A*" detected in the Gene Ontology as an example. The domain experts believe that "*beta-carotene*" is an antioxidant that converts to vitamin A (which is not an *is-a* relation), while SNOMED CT has an *is-a* relation between "*Beta-carotene (substance)*" and "*Retinol (substance)*" (with a synonym "*Vitamin A*"), indicating that this is an incorrect *is-a* relation in the SNOMED CT. Consider "*Abscess of thumb of left hand (disorder)*" *is-a* "*Abscess of finger of left hand (disorder)*" detected in the SNOMED CT. It was obtained by leveraging an existing relation "*Thumb*" *is-a* "*Finger*" in both UWDA and FMA. However, the detected missing *is-a* relation is invalid since, in

SNOMED CT "*Finger*" only includes the second to fifth digit of the hand (i.e., "*Thumb*" is not a "*Finger*").

6.3.3 Discussion About the Approach and Potential Directions

Distinction with Related Work

Other auditing methods designed for a specific terminology including pattern-based, lexical-based, and deep learning-based methods usually rely on the knowledge in the terminology itself and require transferring knowledge to features for representing concepts in order to identify missing *is-a* relations between concepts [112, 113]. Therefore, the effectiveness of such methods to some extent relies on the terminology itself (i.e., internal knowledge), while this method leverages both internal and external knowledge through the UMLS to perform the auditing. More importantly, this method enables the auditing of multiple source terminologies at the same time.

Limitations and Future Work

In this study, we only evaluated the SNOMED CT and Gene Ontology due to the lack of expertise in other terminologies. Although the evaluation results showed that our transformation-based method is effective in identifying missing *is-a* relations in the SNOMED CT and Gene Ontology, additional evaluation by domain experts is still needed to assess the effectiveness of our method for auditing other source terminologies. Another limitation of this approach is regarding the incorrect *is-a* relations that can be further revealed through manual examination of the invalid missing *is-a* relations identified by our method. It would be desirable to develop an automated approach to detect such incorrect *is-a* relations in the source terminologies.

Conclusions: In this section, we introduced a transformation-based auditing method to detect potentially missing *is-a* relations in the UMLS source terminologies. Leveraging rich knowledge in the UMLS (2019AB release), our method is able to audit multiple terminologies at the same time. Experts' evaluation showed the effectiveness of our method. Since the source terminologies are regularly integrated into the UMLS, quality improvement of its source terminologies will directly enhance the quality of the UMLS itself.

6.4   Enriched Lexical Attributes

In this section, we discuss a lexical-based approach for automatic and exhaustive detection of potentially missing *is-a* relations in SNOMED CT. We model each concept with an enriched set of lexical features, which leverages words and noun phrases not only in the name of the concept itself but also in the names of the concept's ancestors. Then we perform subset inclusion checking for concept pairs that are not present in the existing inferred *is-a* hierarchy. Each subset inclusion relation identified is a potentially missing *is-a* relation detected. A random sample of detected missing *is-a* relations is reviewed by a domain expert to evaluate the effectiveness of our approach.

6.4.1   Main Steps of the Enriched Lexical Attributes Method

The September 2017 release of SNOMED CT (US edition) is used for the tasks discussed in this section. We perform three main steps for exhaustive detection of potentially missing *is-a* relations in SNOMED CT: (1) identify a list of stop words/phrases and antonym pairs which may lead to incorrect suggestion of missing *is-a* relations; (2) construct a set of lexical features for each concept by leveraging the words and noun phrases in the concept itself as well as in its ancestors; and (3) check the subset inclusions between each candidate pair of concepts to suggest potentially missing *is-a* relations.

Identifying Stop Words/Phrases and Antonym Pairs

Stop words/phrases may result in wrongly suggested missing *is-a* relations (or false positives). Take concepts *"Velopharyngeal incompetence due to cleft palate (disorder)"* and *"Cleft palate (disorder)"* as an example, even though the set of lexical features of the former concept contains that of the latter concept, there should not be an *is-a* relation between these two concepts. Words/phrases such as "due to" are highly likely to suggest false positives and thus are considered as stop words/phrases. Therefore, we leveraged a list of stop words/phrases used in Sect. 5.3, including: "and," "or," "no," "not," "without," "due to," "secondary to," "except," "by," "after," "co-occurrent," "bilateral," "examination," "able," "amputation," "removal," "replacement," "resection," "excision," "reaction to," "unable," "failure," "failed," "abnormal," "excluding," "non," and "pre."

Similarly, concept pairs whose lexical features contain antonym pairs are likely to generate erroneous suggestions. For instance, considering concepts *"Secondary malignant neoplasm of right upper lobe of lung (disorder)"* and *"Neoplasm of right lower lobe of lung (disorder)"*, apparently there should not be an *is-a* relation between these two concepts, since the former concept is related to "right upper lobe of lung" while the latter concept is related to "right lower lobe of lung." However, if the former concept inherited a lexical feature "lower" from one of its ancestors, *"Malignant neoplasm of lower respiratory tract (disorder)"*, then the lexical feature set of the former would subsume that of the latter, as a result of which an incorrect *is-a* between the former and latter would be suggested. To collect such potential antonym pairs, we adopted a list of adjective antonym pairs from WordNet [107], including ("open," "closed"), ("acute," "chronic"), ("right," "left"), etc. We also identified additional antonym pairs which are not included in WordNet, such as ("upper," "lower").

Constructing Lexical Features for Concepts

Most existing lexical-based methods for identification of missing *is-a* relations use words in concept names as the lexical features of concepts. In this approach, we model concepts not only using words but also utilizing noun phrases. For each concept, we first preprocess its FSN and identify an initial set of lexical features consisting of words and noun phrases in the concept's FSN. Then we enrich the set with more lexical features inherited from the concept's ancestors.

Preprocessing FSNs of Concepts

We first preprocess the FSNs of concepts before the initialization of lexical feature sets. For each concept, we split its FSN (by space) into words sequentially and remove its semantic tag (e.g., "(disorder)"). The semantic tag will be leveraged while suggesting potentially missing *is-a* relations. We further process special symbols in FSNs such as removing parentheses and square brackets, and replacing backslash with "or" if the FSN does not contain numbers (e.g., "Sickness/injury care" will result in "Sickness or injury care," while "5 mg/ml" will remain intact).

Initializing Lexical Feature Sets with Noun Phrases and Words

In this work, instead of purely using the bag-of-words model, we consider noun phrases as meaningful features of concepts to facilitate the identification of missing *is-a* relations. Take two concepts "*Acute sensitivity to pain (finding)*" and "*Acute pain (finding)*" as an example, if we simply used the bag-of-words model, their lexical feature sets would be {acute, sensitivity, to, pain} and {acute, pain} respectively, where {acute, sensitivity, to, pain} is a superset of {acute, pain} (i.e., more detailed), and thus "*Acute sensitivity to pain (finding)*" would be suggested as a subtype of "*Acute pain (finding)*." However, this suggestion is incorrect since "*Acute sensitivity to pain*" is a finding of pain threshold, while "*Acute pain*" is a finding of a pattern of pain, and there should not be any subsumption relations between these two concepts. The reason for this incorrect suggestion is that the adjective "acute" is the modifier for two different nouns ("sensitivity" and "pain") in these two concepts. To avoid such situations, we model a concept's name as a set of noun phrases and words, where a noun phrase groups the modifier(s) and the corresponding noun as a single feature. Hence in the above example, the two concepts' lexical features will become {acute, sensitivity, to, pain, acute sensitivity} and {acute, pain, acute pain}, which do not have any subset-superset relation.

We use Stanford CoreNLP Parser [126] to identify noun phrases. Note that the parser may recognize noun phrases in different levels of granularity. For instance, for concept *"Anesthesia for procedure on veins of lower leg (procedure)"*, there is a base level noun phrase "lower leg" which is a component of a higher level noun phrase "veins of lower leg." In this work, we only consider the base level noun phrases. That is, we model a concept's FSN initially as a set of individual word(s) and base level noun phrase(s). In this example, the initial set of lexical features for the concept is {anesthesia, for, procedure, on, veins, of, lower, leg, lower leg}.

Enriching Lexical Feature Sets

We enrich concepts' lexical features in two steps. In the first step, for each concept c, we check if its FSN contains noun phrase(s) identified in the initial feature sets of other concepts which are not hierarchically linked with c; and if yes, we add such noun phrase(s) into c's initial lexical feature set. We denote concept c's set of lexical features obtained after the first-step enrichment process as E_{1c}. In the second step, for each concept, we further enrich its set of lexical features with its ancestors' sets of lexical features. It is intuitive that if concept x is a subtype of concept y, then the lexical features or attributes of concept y are also considered to be true for concept x (i.e., x inherits y's attributes). In this work, we maintain a directed graph which is constructed using all the inferred hierarchical *is-a* relations in SNOMED CT, compute its transitive closure, and obtain the ancestors of concepts using the breadth-first search. While performing the second-step enrichment process for a concept c, if an ancestor a contains stop word(s)/phrase(s), then we do not add a's set of lexical features to c's. More formally, we have

$$E_{2c} = E_{1c} \cup (\bigcup \{E_{1a} \mid a \in A_c \text{ and } a \text{ does not contain any stop words/phrases}\}),$$

where E_{2c} denotes concept c's set of lexical features after the second-step enrichment process, and A_c is the set of c's ancestors.

Table 6.5 shows an example of the initial and enriched sets of lexical features for a concept c: *"Primary malignant neoplasm of cecum (disorder)"* (371977004). The noun phrase identified in the initial set of lexical features is "primary malignant neoplasm" (underlined). After the first-step enrichment (E_{1c}), a new noun phrase "malignant neoplasm" is identified from concepts which are not hierarchically linked with c. After the second-step enrichment (E_{2c}), more noun phrases and words are inherited from c's ancestors. For instance, noun phrase "large intestine" is inherited from the initial lexical feature set of c's parent – *"Primary malignant neoplasm of large intestine (disorder)"* and noun phrase "malignant tumor" is inherited from c's other parent—*"Malignant tumor of cecum (disorder)."*

Table 6.5 The initial and enriched sets of lexical features of an example concept c: *Primary malignant neoplasm of cecum (disorder)* (371977004). Noun phrases are underlined

c's FSN	Primary malignant neoplasm of cecum (disorder)
Initial set	{primary, malignant, neoplasm, of, cecum, primary malignant neoplasm}
Enriched set E_{1c}	{primary, malignant, neoplasm, of, cecum, primary malignant neoplasm, malignant neoplasm}
Enriched set E_{2c}	{primary, malignant, neoplasm, of, cecum, primary malignant neoplasm, malignant neoplasm, abdominal, mass, abdominal mass, disorder, digestive, structure, digestive structure, finding, large, intestine, large intestine, neoplastic, disease, neoplastic disease, malignant neoplastic disease, viscus, structure finding, body, region, body region, trunk, trunk structure, abdomen, tumor, malignant tumor, organ, digestive organ, gastrointestinal, tract, gastrointestinal tract, system, digestive system, intraabdominal, intraabdominal organ, bowel, bowel finding, lower, lower gastrointestinal tract, body system, abdominal organ finding, abdominal organ, gastrointestinal tract finding, segment, abdominal segment, intestinal, intestinal tract, digestive system finding, system finding, body structure, digestive tract, cecal, cecal mass}

6.4.2   Identifying Potentially Missing is-a Relations

To automatically suggest potentially missing *is-a* relations, we first produce candidate pairs of concepts (say x and y) which meet the following conditions:

- concepts x and y are within the same sub-hierarchy (we assume that concepts in different sub-hierarchies do not have hierarchical *is-a* relations since sub-hierarchies in SNOMED CT do not share common concepts);
- x and y are not hierarchically linked through existing *is-a* relations;
- x and y share the same semantic tag;
- neither x nor y contains any stop word/phrase; and
- the enriched sets of lexical features E_{2x} and E_{2y} do not contain antonym pairs.

Then for each candidate pair of concepts (x, y), we systematically compare their enriched sets of lexical features E_{2x} and E_{2y} as follows: if E_{2x} is a superset of E_{2y}, then "concept x *is-a* concept y" will be suggested as a potentially missing *is-a* relation; if E_{2x} is a subset of E_{2y}, then "concept y *is-a* concept x" will be suggested as a potentially missing *is-a* relation; otherwise, nothing will be suggested.

Since our suggestion of missing *is-a* relations is in an exhaustive way, it may result in redundant missing *is-a* relations A missing *is-a* relation concept x *is-a* concept y is considered to be redundant if,

- there exist a concept z such that "concept x *is-a* concept z" is a suggested missing relation and y is an ancestor of z; and
- there exist a concept s such that "concept s *is-a* concept y" is a suggested missing relation and s is an ancestor of x.

6.4.3   Potential Missing *is-a* Relations Identified

This approach was applied to all the sub-hierarchies of SNOMED CT except "*SNOMED CT Model Component (metadata)*" (e.g., definition status) and "*Special concept (special concept)*" (e.g., inactive concept). A total of 38,615 potentially missing hierarchical is-a relations were suggested. For detailed results, please see [127].

6.4.4   Domain Expert Evaluation

To evaluate the effectiveness of our approach for detecting missing *is-a* relations, we randomly selected a sample of 100 potentially missing *is-a* relations from the "*Clinical finding*" sub-hierarchy. A domain expert reviewed the sample and verified that 90 out of 100 missing *is-a* relations are valid (or true positives), indicating that our approach achieved a precision of 90%.

For each false positive (i.e., invalid missing *is-a* relation suggested), we provided the domain expert with the existing *is-a* relation(s), which lead to the suggestion of the false positive. The domain expert further reviewed these existing *is-a* relations and checked whether any of them is problematic.

Analysis of False Positive Cases

We manually examined the false positive cases for potential causes. For instance, our approach suggests a false positive: "*Familial malignant neoplasm of pancreas (disorder)*" *is-a* "*Malignant tumor of body of pancreas (disorder)*," since the former concept inherits a lexical feature "body" from its ancestor "*Mass of body region (finding).*" However, the meaning of "body" in "*Malignant tumor of body of pancreas (disorder)*" is different than its meaning in "*Mass of body region (finding).*" The former refers to the finding site of structure of body of pancreas, while the latter refers to the finding site of body region structure. Therefore, there should not be an *is-a* relation between the two concepts. In this case, the false positive is due to the varied meanings of a word in a different context.

Another cause of false positives is the incorrect existing *is-a* relations in SNOMED CT that our approach leverages to suggest potentially missing *is-a* relations. For instance, our approach suggests *"Encysted hydrocele of spermatic cord (disorder)" is-a "Soft tissue lesion of pelvic region (disorder),"* which is incorrect since hydrocele refers to a small "bag of fluid" and is not considered as a soft tissue lesion. This incorrect suggestion is due to an existing relation: *"Encysted hydrocele of spermatic cord (disorder)" is-a "Soft tissue lesion (disorder)"*. In addition, there are two false positives caused by the same existing relation: *"Algodystrophy (disorder) is-a "Degenerative disorder (disorder)"* in the September 2017 release of SNOMED CT US edition that we used. It is worth noting that this relation is no longer existent in the current version of SNOMED CT.

6.4.5   Analysis of the Approach

In this section, we introduce a lexical approach for exhaustive detection of potentially missing hierarchical *is-a* relations in SNOMED CT. It can be seen that our approach can not only detect intuitive/straightforward relations such as *"Primary adenosquamous cell carcinoma of larynx (disorder)" is-a "Carcinoma of larynx (disorder),"* but also uncover complicated cases such as *"Genital herpes simplex (disorder)" is-a "Infectious disease of genitourinary system (disorder)"* and *"Plasmodium vivax malaria with rupture of spleen (disorder)" is-a "Infectious disease of abdomen (disorder)."* Since our approach only requires the hierarchical *is-a* structure and concept names as the input, it can be generally applied to other terminologies or ontologies.

Comparison with Previous Work

In Sect. 5.3, we discussed a structural-lexical approach for the detection of potentially missing *is-a* relations in SNOMED CT, by leveraging the lexical attributes of concepts in non-lattice subgraphs. In this work, we perform exhaustive detection of potentially missing *is-a* relations without limiting to the non-lattice substructures. More importantly, this work identifies previously undiscovered missing *is-a* relations. Among 38,615 potentially missing *is-a* relations identified in this work, 36,534 (94.6%) are newly discovered compared with those in Sect. 5.3. Among 6,946 potentially missing *is-a* relations from the *Clinical finding* sub-hierarchy in this work, 6,081 (87.5%) are newly identified compared with those in Sect. 5.3.

Another major distinction is regarding the construction of lexical features for concepts. In Sect. 5.3, a concept in a non-lattice subgraph is modeled as a set of words in its FSN with enriched lexical features inherited from its ancestors within the non-lattice subgraph. In this work, we model each concept as a set of words and noun phrases, with enriched lexical features inherited from all its ancestors in the entire SNOMED CT.

Limitations and Future Work

Although the results showed that this approach is effective in identifying missing hierarchical *is-a* relations, there still remains several limitations.

Our evaluation is limited in that it only involved samples from the *Clinical Finding* sub-hierarchy. Manual review of the detected missing *is-a* relations by domain experts is time-consuming and labor-intensive. In future work, we plan to investigate methods that leverage external knowledge (e.g., external ontologies, biomedical literature) to automatically identify supporting evidence for the detected missing *is-a* relations to relieve the manual burden.

In addition, our approach relies on the Stanford CoreNLP Parser to identify noun phrases in the concept names. However, sometimes the Stanford Parser may not accurately recognize noun phrases. For instance, for concept *"Gluthathione peroxidase deficiency (disorder),"* it recognizes "peroxidase deficiency" as a noun phrase. However, "Gluthathione peroxidase" is a more meaningful noun phrase to serve as a lexical feature for this concept.

Conclusions: In this section, we presented a lexical-based approach to exhaustively detect potentially missing hierarchical *is-a* relations in SNOMED CT. For each concept, a set of enriched lexical features consisting of words and noun phrases in the name of the concept itself and its ancestors is identified. Pairwise comparison of the concepts' lexical features automatically suggested potentially missing *is-a* relations.

6.5   Evidence-Based Method

In this section, we introduce a novel evidence-based approach for uncovering missing relations and erroneous existing relations in GO (including but not limited to *is-a* relations). The basic idea of the approach is leveraging lexical patterns exhibited in related concept pairs (i.e., existing relations) in GO to identify potentially missing relations between unrelated concept pairs. We represent each GO concept's name with a sequence of words along with part-of-speech tags. Such representation enables us to automatically generate lexical patterns from related concept pairs, serving as the first layer evidence to suggest potentially missing relations between unrelated concept pairs. For each suggested missing relation, we further identify a concept quadruple consisting of concepts in two existing relations as the second layer of evidence, which resembles the difference among the concept quadruple consisting of concepts in the missing relation and the existing relation based on which the missing relation is suggested.

6.5.1 Obtaining Dual-Layer Evidence

Concept Name Representation

Given a concept C in GO, we represent its concept name as a sequence of words $W(C) = [w_1, w_2, w_3, \ldots, w_n]$ along with a sequence of part-of-speech tags $T(C) = [t_1, t_2, t_3, \ldots, t_n]$ corresponding to each word, where n is the number of words in the concept name, $w_i (1 \leq i \leq n)$ is the i-th word in the concept name, and $t_i (1 \leq i \leq n)$ is the part-of-speech tag of w_i. For instance, GO concept $C =$ "*nitric oxide biosynthetic process*" (GO:0006809) can be represented as

$$W(C) = [\text{"}nitric\text{"}, \text{"}oxide\text{"}, \text{"}biosynthetic\text{"}, \text{"}process\text{"}],$$
$$T(C) = [ADJ, NOUN, ADJ, NOUN].$$

For the part-of-speech tagging, we used the English transformer pipeline of the open source natural language processing (NLP) library spaCy [114].

Computing Related Concept Pairs

GO concepts are connected with various relationships including *is-a*, *part-of*, *has-part*, *regulates*, *negatively-regulates*, and *positively-regulates* [128, 129]. A related concept pair is a pair of concepts that are directly or indirectly connected with a relationship. To obtain all the related concept pairs in GO, we first extract directly related concept pairs using the GOATOOLS python library [130], and then obtain indirectly related concept pairs by computing transitive closure leveraging the reasoning rules given in Table 6.6. For example, one of the reasoning rules is that if A *is-a* B and B *part-of* C, then it can be inferred A *part-of* C. Note that these inference rules may involve more complex cases combining multiple rules. For instance, if A *is-a* B, B *part-of* C, and C *is-a* D, then it can be inferred A *part-of* D using the reasoning rules (2) and (7) in Table 6.6.

Algorithm 1: The algorithm to compute all the concepts that a given concept C directly or indirectly connects to via *is-a*.

---

1 **procedure** *isa(C)*:
2 $\quad$ **Initialization**:
3 $\quad$ direct *is-a* parents $D \leftarrow$ direct parents of C
4 $\quad$ all *is-a* ancestors $S \leftarrow D$
5 $\quad$ **for** d *in* D **do**
6 $\quad\quad$ | S.add(*isa(d)*)   ▷ Recursive call
7 $\quad$ **end**
8 $\quad$ **return** S

Table 6.6 Gene Ontology reasoning rules for relationships *is-a*, *part-of*, *has-part*, *regulates*, *negatively-regulates* (*n-regulates*), and *positively-regulates* (*p-regulates*) [128, 129]

Relationship	Reasoning rules	
is-a	(1) *A is-a B, B is-a C*	$\Rightarrow$ *A is-a C*
	(2) *A is-a B, B part-of C*	$\Rightarrow$ *A part-of C*
	(3) *A is-a B, B has-part C*	$\Rightarrow$ *A has-part C*
	(4) *A is-a B, B regulates C*	$\Rightarrow$ *A regulates C*
	(5) *A is-a B, B n-regulates C*	$\Rightarrow$ *A n-regulates C*
	(6) *A is-a B, B p-regulates C*	$\Rightarrow$ *A p-regulates C*
part-of	(7) *A part-of B, B is-a C*	$\Rightarrow$ *A part-of C*
	(8) *A part-of B, B part-of C*	$\Rightarrow$ *A part-of C*
has-part	(9) *A has-part B, B is-a C*	$\Rightarrow$ *A has-part C*
	(10) *A has-part B, B has-part C*	$\Rightarrow$ *A has-part C*
regulates	(11) *A regulates B, B is-a C*	$\Rightarrow$ *A regulates C*
	(12) *A regulates B, B regulates C*	$\Rightarrow$ *A regulates C*
n-regulates	(13) *A n-regulates B, B is-a C*	$\Rightarrow$ *A n-regulates C*
p-regulates	(14) *A p-regulates B, B is-a C*	$\Rightarrow$ *A p-regulates C*
	(15) *A p-regulates B, B p-regulates C*	$\Rightarrow$ *A p-regulates C*
	(16) *A n-regulates B, B n-regulates C*	$\Rightarrow$ *A p-regulates C*

Given a concept C, Algorithm 1 presents our procedure to obtain all the concepts that C connects to via the *is-a* relationship; and Algorithm 2 demonstrates how to compute all the concepts that C connects to via the *part-of* relationship. The concept pairs connected via other relationships can be similarly obtained. Note that such transitive closure for a given concept can be obtained through GOATOOLS (or other tools such as Owlready2 and OWL API) for the *is-a* relationship, but not for other relationships.

Algorithm 2: The algorithm to compute all the concepts that a given concept C directly or indirectly connects to via *part-of*.

1 **procedure** *partof*(C):
2   **Initialization:**
3   direct *is-a* parents $D \leftarrow$ direct parents of C
4   direct *part-of* values $E \leftarrow$ direct *part-of* values of C
5   all *part-of* values $S \leftarrow E$
6   **for** d in D **do**
7 | S.add(*partof*(d))   ▷ Recursive call
8   **end**
9   **for** e in E **do**
10 | S.add(*partof*(e))   ▷ Recursive call
11 | S.add(*isa*(e))   ▷ Calling *isa*
12   **end**
13   **Return** S

Extracting Lexical Patterns from Concept Pairs

We extract lexical patterns from pairs of concepts having at least one word in common. Given a pair of concepts (C_1, C_2) with

$$W(C_1) = [w_{(1,1)}, w_{(1,2)}, w_{(1,3)}, \ldots, w_{(1,p)}],$$
$$W(C_2) = [w_{(2,1)}, w_{(2,2)}, w_{(2,3)}, \ldots, w_{(2,q)}],$$

such that C_1 and C_2 have a set of common words $K = \{k_i \mid 1 \leq i \leq s\}$, where s is the total number of commons words, we can generate a lexical pattern of (C_1, C_2):

$$L(C_1, C_2) = (W'(C_1), W'(C_2)),$$

where $W'(C_1)$ is obtained by replacing each common word k_i in $W(C_1)$ with an abstract label K_i, and $W'(C_2)$ is obtained by replacing each common word k_i in $W(C_2)$ with K_i.

For instance, considering the following two concepts in Fig. 6.11(1):

$$A = \text{``\textit{nitric oxide biosynthetic process}''} \ (\text{GO:0006809}),$$
$$B = \text{``\textit{cellular nitrogen compound biosynthetic process}''}$$
$$(\text{GO:0044271}),$$

they have two words in common, that is, $K = \{\text{``\textit{biosynthetic},''} \ \text{``\textit{process}''}\}$. After replacing "*biosynthetic*" with K_1 and "*process*" with K_2, the obtained lexical pattern is:

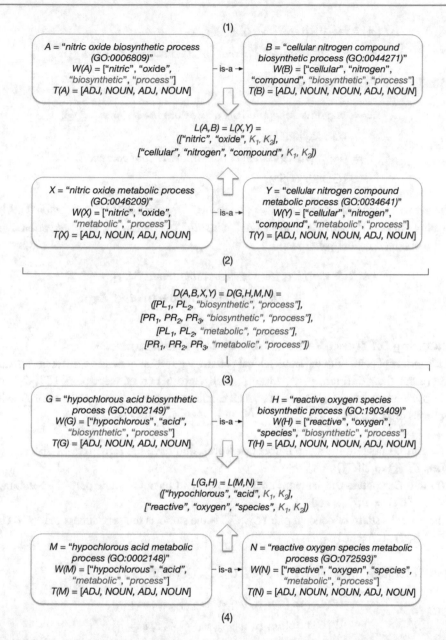

Fig. 6.11 (1) Existing *is-a* relation between concept $A =$ "*nitric oxide biosynthetic process*" (GO:0006809) and $B =$ "*cellular nitrogen compound biosynthetic process*" (GO:0044271) that is leveraged to generate the lexical pattern $L(A, B)$; (2) Missing *is-a* relation (arrow in red) between concept $X =$ "*nitric oxide metabolic process*" (GO:0046209) and concept $Y =$ "*cellular nitrogen compound metabolic process*" (GO:0034641) with the same lexical pattern; (3) and (4): Pair of existing *is-a* relations that resembles the difference between (1) and (2)

$$L(A, B) =([\text{``}nitric\text{''}, \text{``}oxide\text{''}, K_1, K_2],$$
$$[\text{``}cellular\text{''}, \text{``}nitrogen\text{''}, \text{``}compound\text{''}, K_1, K_2]).$$

Similarly, in Fig. 6.12(1), for concepts

$$X = \text{``}negative\ regulation\ of\ corticosterone\ secretion\text{''}$$
$$(\text{GO:2000853}),$$
$$Y = \text{``}negative\ regulation\ of\ mineralocorticoid\ secretion\text{''}$$
$$(\text{GO:2000856}),$$

they have four common words (i.e., $K = \{\text{``}negative,\text{''} \text{``}regulation,\text{''} \text{``}of,\text{''} \text{``}secretion\text{''}\}$). After replacing "*negative*" with K_1, "*regulation*" with K_2, "*of*" with K_3, and "*secretion*" with K_4, the obtained lexical pattern is:

$$L(X, Y) =([K_1, K_2, K_3, \text{``}corticosterone, \text{''}K_4],$$
$$[K_1, K_2, K_3, \text{``}mineralocorticoid, \text{''}K_4]).$$

Generating Difference Patterns from Concept Quadruples

For two concept pairs with the same lexical pattern, we further generate a difference pattern to represent their different parts. More formally, given two concept pairs (C_1, C_2) and (C_3, C_4), we consider (C_1, C_2, C_3, C_4) as a candidate concept quadruple if the following conditions are met:

1. C_1 and C_3 contain the same number of words, and have the same part-of-speech tags, i.e., $T(C_1) = T(C_3)$;
2. C_2 and C_4 contain the same number of words, and have the same part-of-speech tags, i.e., $T(C_2) = T(C_4)$; and
3. the lexical pattern of concept pair (C_1, C_2) is the same as that of concept pair (C_3, C_4), i.e., $L(C_1, C_2) = L(C_3, C_4)$.

For a candidate concept quadruple (C_1, C_2, C_3, C_4) with

$$W(C_1) = [w_{(1,1)}, w_{(1,2)}, w_{(1,3)}, \ldots, w_{(1,p)}],$$
$$W(C_2) = [w_{(2,1)}, w_{(2,2)}, w_{(2,3)}, \ldots, w_{(2,q)}],$$
$$W(C_3) = [w_{(3,1)}, w_{(3,2)}, w_{(3,3)}, \ldots, w_{(3,p)}],$$
$$W(C_4) = [w_{(4,1)}, w_{(4,2)}, w_{(4,3)}, \ldots, w_{(4,q)}],$$

we can generate a difference pattern:

$$D(C_1, C_2, C_3, C_4) = (W^*(C_1), W^*(C_2), W^*(C_3), W^*(C_4)),$$

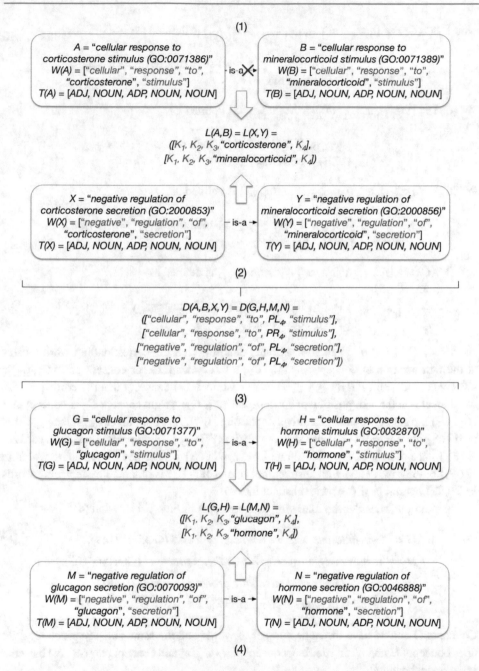

Fig. 6.12 (1) Erroneous existing *is-a* relation (red cross) between concept $A =$ "*cellular response to corticosterone stimulus*" (GO:0071386) and concept $B =$ "*cellular response to mineralocorticoid stimulus*" (GO:0071389) that is leveraged to generate the lexical pattern $L(A, B)$; (2) Invalid missing *is-a* relation between *GO:2000853* and *GO:2000856* with the same lexical pattern; (3) and (4): Pair of existing *is-a* relations that resembles the difference between (1) and (2)

where $W^*(C_1) = [w^*_{(1,1)}, w^*_{(1,2)}, w^*_{(1,3)}, \ldots, w^*_{(1,p)}]$ is defined as:

$$w^*_{(1,i)} = \begin{cases} w_{(1,i)}, & \text{if } \exists j(1 \leq j \leq q) \text{ such that } w_{(1,i)} = w_{(2,j)}, \\ PL_i, & \text{otherwise;} \end{cases}$$

$W^*(C_2) = [w^*_{(2,1)}, w^*_{(2,2)}, w^*_{(2,3)}, \ldots, w^*_{(2,q)}]$ is defined as:

$$w^*_{(2,j)} = \begin{cases} w_{(2,j)}, & \text{if } \exists i(1 \leq i \leq p) \text{ such that } w_{(2,j)} = w_{(1,i)}, \\ PR_j, & \text{otherwise;} \end{cases}$$

$W^*(C_3) = [w^*_{(3,1)}, w^*_{(3,2)}, w^*_{(3,3)}, \ldots, w^*_{(3,p)}]$ is defined as:

$$w^*_{(3,i)} = \begin{cases} w_{(3,i)}, & \text{if } \exists j(1 \leq j \leq q) \text{ such that } w_{(3,i)} = w_{(4,j)}, \\ PL_i, & \text{otherwise;} \end{cases}$$

and $W^*(C_4) = [w^*_{(4,1)}, w^*_{(4,2)}, w^*_{(4,3)}, \ldots, w^*_{(4,q)}]$ is defined as:

$$w^*_{(4,j)} = \begin{cases} w_{(4,j)}, & \text{if } \exists i(1 \leq i \leq p) \text{ such that } w_{(4,j)} = w_{(3,i)}, \\ PR_j, & \text{otherwise.} \end{cases}$$

Here PL_i $(1 \leq i \leq p)$ is an abstract label denoting that the corresponding word locates at the i-th position of concept pair (C_1, C_2)'s left concept C_1 or concept pair (C_3, C_4)'s left concept C_3; and $PR_j(1 \leq j \leq q)$ is an abstract label denoting that the corresponding word locates at the j-th position of concept pair (C_1, C_2)'s right concept C_2 or concept pair (C_3, C_4)'s right concept C_4. Intuitively speaking, $W^*(C_1)$ is obtained by replacing words in $W(C_1)$ but not in $W(C_2)$ with abstract labels; $W^*(C_2)$ is obtained by replacing words in $W(C_2)$ but not in $W(C_1)$ with abstract labels; $W^*(C_3)$ is obtained by replacing words in $W(C_3)$ but not in $W(C_4)$ with abstract labels; and $W^*(C_4)$ is obtained by replacing words in $W(C_4)$ but not in $W(C_3)$ with abstract labels.

For example, consider the following four concepts in Figs. 6.11(3) and (4):

G = "*hypochlorous acid biosynthetic process*" (GO:0002149),

H = "*reactive oxygen species biosynthetic process*" (GO:1903409),

M = "*hypochlorous acid metabolic process*" (GO:0002148),

N = "*reactive oxygen species metabolic process*" (GO:0072593).

Concepts G and M have the same number of words and the same part-of-speech tags. So does concepts H and N. In addition, concept pair (G, H) and concept pair (M, N) have the same lexical pattern:

$$(["hypochlorous", "acid", "K_1, K_2],$$
$$["reactive", "oxygen", "species, "K_1, K_2]).$$

Therefore, (G, H, M, N) forms a candidate concept quadruple. For concept G, since words "*hypochlorous*" and "*acid*" do not appear in H, they are replaced by labels PL_1 and PL_2 respectively, resulting in $W^*(G) = [PL_1, PL_2, "biosynthetic", "process"]$; for concept H, since words "*reactive*", "*oxygen*", and "*species*" does not appear in G, they are replaced by labels PR_1, PR_2, and PR_3 respectively, resulting in $W^*(H) = [PR_1, PR_2, PR_3, "biosynthetic", "process"]$; and similarly, we can obtain $W^*(M) = [PL_1, PL_2, "metabolic", "process"]$ and $W^*(N) = [PR_1, PR_2, PR_3, "metabolic", "process"]$. Therefore, the difference pattern of (G, H, M, N) is:

$$D(G, H, M, N) =$$
$$([PL_1, PL_2, "biosynthetic", "process"],$$
$$[PR_1, PR_2, PR_3, "biosynthetic", "process"],$$
$$[PL_1, PL_2, "metabolic", "process"],$$
$$[PR_1, PR_2, PR_3, "metabolic", "process"]).$$

Note that the difference pattern represents the difference between two pairs of concepts. In this example, we can see that the different parts are ["*biosynthetic*", "*process*"] in concept pair (G, H) and ["*metabolic*", "*process*"] in concept pair (M, N).

Evidence-Based Identification of Relational Defects

We focus on identifying relational defects regarding the following set of GO relationships: $R = \{is\text{-}a, part\text{-}of, has\text{-}part, regulates, negatively\text{-}regulates, positively\text{-}regulates\}$. For each relationship $r \in R$, we extract lexical patterns for all the related concept pairs connected via r. Then we generate difference patterns for candidate concept quadruples (C_1, C_2, C_3, C_4) where (C_1, C_2) and (C_3, C_4) are related concept pairs connected via r. We leverage these lexical patterns and difference patterns as two layers of evidence to identify potentially missing r relations as follows.

Given a pair of concepts X and Y that are not related via any GO relationship, if

1. there exists a related concept pair (A, B) connected via r, such that

$$L(X, Y) = L(A, B),$$

and
2. there exists a candidate concept quadruple (G, H, M, N) where (G, H) and (M, N) are related concept pairs connected via r, such that

$$D(A, B, X, Y) = D(G, H, M, N),$$

then we suggest a potentially missing r relation between concepts X and Y. Here the related concept pair (A, B) serves as the first layer of evidence, and the concept quadruple

(G, H, M, N) serves as the second layer of evidence. Note that a potentially missing relation may be derived by multiple first and second layers of evidence.

More specifically, for concepts A and B, given that they have common words and are related via r, we assume that the different words between A and B are highly likely to make their r relation hold, which is leveraged as the first layer of evidence for suggesting an r relation between concepts X and Y, because (X, Y) have the same lexical pattern as (A, B) (i.e., the different words between X and Y are the same as the different words between A and B). For instance, for concept $A = $ "*nitric oxide biosynthetic process*" (GO:0006809) and concept $B = $ "*cellular nitrogen compound biosynthetic process*" (GO:0044271) in Fig. 6.11(1) related by *is-a*, we assume that "*nitric oxide*" in A and "*cellular nitrogen compound*" in B are highly likely to make the *is-a* relation hold; and this serves as the first layer of evidence for us to suggest a potentially missing *is-a* relation between concept $X = $ "*nitric oxide metabolic process*" (GO:0046209) and concept $Y = $ "*cellular nitrogen compound metabolic process*" (GO:0034641) in Fig. 6.11(2).

Although concept pair (X, Y) have the same lexical pattern as concept pair (A, B), the common words of A and B are distinct from that of X and Y. Therefore, we seek further evidence of such distinction among other related r concept pairs in candidate concept quadruples (i.e., difference pattern). For the above example (A, B, X, Y) in Figs. 6.11(1) and (2), the difference pattern is "*biosynthetic process*" versus "*metabolic process*;" and there exists a candidate concept quadruple (G, H, M, N) where (G, H) and (M, N) are related *is-a* concept pairs (see Figs. 6.11(3) and (4)), such that (G, H, M, N) have the same difference pattern ("*biosynthetic process*" versus "*metabolic process*"), the second layer of evidence.

Note that in some instances, the same lexical pattern could be obtained through different relationship types. We discard such patterns as they would suggest multiple types of missing relations among the same two concepts (e.g., A *is-a* B and A *part-of* B both being suggested), which is unlikely to be true.

In addition, it is possible that a suggested missing relation can be inferred by other suggested missing relations and existing GO relations using the reasoning rules in Table 6.6. To identify such cases, we check whether each suggested missing relation is included in the transitive closure computed with all the other suggested missing relations and existing relations in GO. Such suggestions are redundant and hence removed. For example, consider the following two suggestions for the missing relationships: (1) *regulates* relation between concepts "*regulation of NK T cell differentiation*" (GO:0051136) and "*NK T cell activation*" (GO:0051132); (2) *is-a* relation between the concepts "*regulation of NK T cell differentiation*" (GO:0051136) and "*regulation of NK T cell activation*" (GO:0051133). However, GO currently has the *regulates* relation between concepts: "*regulation of NK T cell activation*" (GO:0051133) and "*NK T cell activation*" (GO:0051132) which together with (2) infers the (1) through reasoning rule 4) in Table 6.6.

For the potentially missing relations automatically suggested by our approach, manual review by domain experts is required to assess their validity. If a suggested missing r relation between concepts X and Y is agreed by domain experts, then it is considered a valid missing relation (e.g., *is-a* relation between *"nitric oxide metabolic process"* and *"cellular nitrogen compound metabolic process"* in Fig. 6.11(2)). However, if a suggested missing r relation between concepts X and Y is disagreed by domain experts, then the concept pair (A, B) that is leveraged as the first layer of evidence to suggest the missing relation is further examined as follows: if the r relation between concepts A and B is agreed by domain experts, then we consider the suggested missing r relation between X and Y is a false positive suggested by our approach; but if the r relation between concepts A and B is disagreed by domain experts, then it is considered as a valid erroneous existing relation.

For instance, Fig. 6.12(2) shows a potentially missing *is-a* relation between concepts $X =$ *"negative regulation of corticosterone secretion"* (GO:2000853) and $Y =$ *"negative regulation of mineralocorticoid secretion"* (GO:2000856) suggested by our approach by leveraging an existing *is-a* relation between concepts $A =$ *"cellular response to corticosterone stimulus"* (GO:0071386) and $B =$ *"cellular response to mineralocorticoid stimulus"* (GO:0071389), as shown in Fig. 6.12(1). However, the suggested *is-a* relation between *"negative regulation of corticosterone secretion"* and *"negative regulation of mineralocorticoid secretion"* is disagreed by domain experts, since mineralocorticoid is considered a subtype of corticosterone (not the other way around) [131]. Further, the *is-a* relation between the evidence concept pair *"cellular response to corticosterone stimulus"* and *"cellular response to mineralocorticoid stimulus"* is also disagreed by domain experts, and thus an erroneous existing *is-a* relation.

Evaluation

To evaluate the effectiveness of our approach, all the potential missing relations obtained are manually reviewed by our local domain experts who have expertise in systems biology and genomics. Any disagreements among the experts are resolved through discussion. For each potentially missing relation, the domain experts are provided with the concept names and web links (in QuickGO [132]) of the two concepts involved in the relation. If a potentially missing relation is confirmed as valid by domain experts, then we consider it as a true missing relation; otherwise, domain experts are further provided with the concept pair that was leveraged as the first layer of evidence to suggest the missing relation. If the evidence concept pair is confirmed to have a valid relation by domain experts, then we consider the original missing relation as a false positive; however, if the evidence concept pair is confirmed to be an invalid relation, then we consider the evidence concept pair as an erroneous existing relation.

6.5.2   Potential Inconsistencies Uncovered and the Evaluation Performed

In this approach, we used the 2021-12-15 release of GO with 50,757 concepts. We focused on auditing the following GO relationships: *is-a*, *part-of*, *has-part*, *regulates*, *negatively-regulates*, and *positively-regulates*.

In total, our approach suggested 2,722 cases of potentially missing relations in GO, among which 1,856 relations can be inferred by others. Removal of such redundant relations resulted in 866 potentially missing relations (702 *is-a*, 144 *part-of*, 19 *regulates*, and 1 *part-of*). Note that the approach suggested only two *negatively-regulates* potential missing relations which were both found to be redundant. The method did not suggest any *positively-regulates* potential missing relations. The 866 potentially missing relations were suggested by 764 unique lexical patterns. Out of these, 688 lexical patterns suggested only one potentially missing relation, while 76 suggested more than one potentially missing relation. Table 6.7 shows ten examples of lexical patterns and the number of potentially missing relations each pattern suggested. For instance, lexical pattern ($[K_1, "differentiation"], [K_1, "activation"]$) was leveraged to suggest five potentially missing *is-a* relations.

Evaluation Results

The entire set of 866 potentially missing relations suggested by this approach was evaluated by local domain experts. Out of 866 potentially missing relations suggested, 821 were identified by local domain experts to be valid missing relations (661 *is-a*, 143 *part-of*, 1 *has-part*, and 16 *regulates*) and 45 revealed valid erroneous existing relations (41 *is-a*, 1 *part-of*, and 3 *regulates*).

Table 6.8 lists 10 examples of valid relational defects in the random sample, including a missing *part-of* relation between "*cardiac right atrium formation*" (GO:0003217) and "*heart formation*" (GO:0060914), and an erroneous *is-a* relation between "*hypochlorous acid metabolic process*" (GO:0002148) and "*organic acid metabolic process*" (GO:0006082).

For a detailed results and analysis, please see [133].

6.5.3   Further Analysis of the Method and the Results

In this section, we introduced an evidence-based approach leveraging automatically extracted lexical patterns to facilitate identification of two types of relational defects in GO: missing relations and erroneous existing relations. A vast majority of potentially missing relations suggested by our approach are *is-a* relations. This is expected as the majority of relations in GO are *is-a* relations. According to local domain experts, 94.8% of potentially missing relations (821 out of 866) are valid missing relations and 5.2% of them (45 out of 866) revealed valid erroneous existing relations. This indicates the effectiveness of our approach

Table 6.7 Ten examples of lexical patterns suggesting the most potentially missing relations and the number of potentially missing relations suggested by each pattern

Lexical pattern	Relationship	No. of potentially missing relations suggested
($[K_1, K_2,$ "import", "across", "plasma", "membrane"], $[K_1, K_2,$ "homeostasis"])	is-a	6
($[K_1, K_2, K_3, K_4,$ "differentiation"], $[K_1, K_2, K_3, K_4,$ "activation"])	is-a	6
(["histone", K_1], ["peptidyl-lysine", K_1])	is-a	5
($[K_1,$ "differentiation"], $[K_1,$ "activation"])	is-a	5
(["dendritic", "cell", K_1], ["lymphocyte", K_1])	is-a	4
($[K_1,$ "dephosphorylation"], $[K_1,$ "modification"])	is-a	4
($[K_1, K_2, K_3, K_4,$ "proliferation"], $[K_1, K_2, K_3, K_4,$ "activation"])	is-a	4
(["N-terminal", $K_1,$ "deamination"], $[K_1,$ "modification"])	is-a	4
($[K_1,$ "activation"], $[K_1,$ "development"])	is-a	3
($[K_1,$ "guanylyltransferase", "activity"], $[K_1,$ "processing"])	is-a	3

that leverages lexical patterns and difference patterns derived from existing GO relations as two layers of evidence.

For the erroneous existing relations identified, considering the *is-a* relation between "*hypochlorous acid metabolic process*" (GO:0002148) and "*organic acid metabolic process*" (GO:0006082), this is invalid since hypochlorous acid is not an organic acid as it does not contain a carbon. Among the 45 erroneous existing relations identified, 7 were *is-a* relations with "*hypochlorous acid metabolic process*" (GO:0002148) as the parent. Local domain experts suggested that some erroneous existing relations may be better represented using a different relationship. For instance, the concepts "*negative regulation of cohesin loading*" (GO:0071923) and "*negative regulation of sister chromatid cohesion*" (GO:0045875) may be better connected through a *part-of* relation than the existing *is-a* relation. There were 16 such cases among the erroneous existing relations identified.

Table 6.8 Ten examples of valid missing relations (M) or erroneous existing relations (E) according to local domain experts

Source concept	Relationship	Target concept	Type
ganglion formation (GO:0061554)	*is-a*	*animal organ formation* (GO:0048645)	M
positive regulation of RIG-I signaling pathway (GO:1900246)	*is-a*	*positive regulation of defense response* (GO:0031349)	M
geranyl diphosphate biosynthetic process (GO:0033384)	*is-a*	*cellular lipid biosynthetic process* (GO:0097384)	M
hypochlorous acid metabolic process (GO:0002148)	*is-a*	*organic acid metabolic process* (GO:0006082)	E
negative regulation of cell septum assembly (GO:1901892)	*is-a*	*negative regulation of cytokinesis* (GO:0032466)	E
cardiac right atrium formation (GO:0003217)	*part-of*	*heart formation* (GO:0060914)	M
endocardial cushion fusion (GO:0003274)	*part-of*	*endocardial cushion formation* (GO:0003272)	M
regulation of cellotriose catabolic process (GO:2000936)	*regulates*	*polysaccharide catabolic process* (GO:0000272)	M
regulation of glycogen catabolic process (GO:0005981)	*regulates*	*glucose catabolic process* (GO:0006007)	M
polyadenylation-dependent ncRNA catabolic process (GO:0043634)	*has-part*	*ncRNA processing* (GO:0034470)	M

Comparison with Related Work

A major difference between this approach and other lexical pattern-based work to audit GO is that the lexical patterns are generated automatically rather than being manually crafted. For instance, in Sect. 6.2, we used three conditional rules (monotonicity, intersection, and sub-concept rules) that were manually defined to uncover missing and erroneous *is-a* relations in GO. Such manual creation of lexical patterns may take extensive exploration of existing concepts and relations of an ontology which is very time-consuming and may require thorough domain knowledge about the ontology. Therefore, automated generation of such patterns from existing relations in the ontology is a considerable improvement in lexical pattern-based ontological auditing. In addition, only *is-a* relations were investigated in Sect. 6.2, while this approach covers a variety of relationships including *is-a*, *part-of*, *has-part*, *regulates*, *negatively-regulates*, and *positively-regulates*. It should also be noted that a vast majority (85.8%) of relational defects identified by this approach is not identifiable by the manually curated rules in Sect. 6.2. Additionally, the local domain expert evaluation in this approach is much more rigorous since the entire set of 866 potentially missing relations suggested by our approach have been assessed. In Sect. 6.2, only a random subset of 210 samples were assessed.

Ontology auditing approaches are discovery oriented in their nature and different approaches are intended to address different types of issues. This makes it harder to compare different approaches in terms of their performance, as there is a lack of gold standard for quality issues in an ontology. However, purely based on the percentage of valid quality issues assessed by local domain experts, our approach outperforms the previous approach using manually crafted lexical patterns in [123], where the monotonicity, intersection, and subconcept rules revealed only 60.61, 60.49, and 46.03% valid quality issues respectively, based on local domain experts' evaluation of 210 instances.

Another advantage of our approach over approaches like the one employed by Agrawal et al. [134], is that the manual effort needed to uncover quality defects is considerably less in our approach. Agrawal et al. approach requires an extensive manual evaluation of the problematic areas of the ontology to locate the exact quality issues. However, this approach directly provides the two concepts where a missing relation may exist and the experts only need to validate whether it is accurate.

GO Consortium Feedback

We have reached out to the GO consortium and submitted our suggested changes as a whole (821 missing relations and 45 erroneous existing relations) for further validation and incorporation to GO. The initial review by the GO editorial team indicated that most of the missing relations and erroneous existing relations we identified seem correct. And they have also independently identified some of the issues we found, and are already working on addressing them, including adding missing axioms for some GO terms, working with external ontology teams (e.g. Chemical Entities of Biological Interest [ChEBI] [135]), and restructuring specific parts of the ontology.

Meanwhile, we have put 20 sample issues (15 missing relations and 5 erroneous existing relations) in the GO-ontology tracking system on GitHub [136]. As of March 10, 2022, 7 issues have received feedback, where 6 of them were agreed by the GO editorial team and revealed different remediation solutions (see Table 6.9). For instance, the missing *part-of* relation between "*bone growth*" (GO:0098868) and "*bone development*"

Table 6.9 Six valid missing relations (M) or erroneous existing relations (E), which were further validated by the GO editorial team and incorporated into GO

Relation	Type	Solution
bone growth (GO:0098868) *part-of* *bone development* (GO:0060348)	M	Relation added
xylan catabolic process (GO:0045493) *is-a* *hemicellulose catabolic process* (GO:2000895)	M	External ontology changed
positive regulation of establishment of turgor in appressorium (GO:0075041) *is-a* *positive regulation of appressorium maturation* (GO:0075037)	M	GO:0075041 obsoleted
purine nucleobase biosynthetic process (GO:0009113) *is-a* *pigment biosynthetic process* (GO:0046148)	E	Relation removed
rhizobactin 1021 biosynthetic process (GO:0019289) *is-a* *catechol-containing compound biosynthetic process* (GO:0009713)	E	Relation removed
positive regulation of prosthetic group metabolic process (GO:0051200) *is-a* *positive regulation of cellular protein metabolic process* (GO:0032270)	E	GO:0051200 obsoleted

(GO:0060348) has been directly added to GO; and the erroneous existing *is-a* relation between "*purine nucleobase biosynthetic process*" (GO:0009113) and "*pigment biosynthetic process*" (GO:0046148) has been directly removed from GO. In the case of the missing *is-*

a relation between "*xylan catabolic process*" (GO:0045493) and "*hemicellulose catabolic process*" (GO:2000895), the issue was found to be a missing *is-a* relation between concepts "*xylan*" (CHEBI:37166) and "*hemicellulose*" (CHEBI:61266) in the external ontology ChEBI that GO reuses. We have reported this missing *is-a* relation to ChEBI (which has been added), and thus the former relation can be inferred in GO.

Note that certain issues uncovered by our approach have helped with identification of additional issues in GO. For instance, while reviewing the missing *is-a* relation between "*positive regulation of establishment of turgor in appressorium*" (GO:0075041) and "*positive regulation of appressorium maturation*" (GO:0075037), the GO editorial team has decided to obsolete not only *GO:0075041*, but also 8 additional concepts including "*regulation of establishment of turgor in appressorium*" (GO:0075040) and "*negative regulation of establishment of turgor in appressorium*" (GO:0075042).

However, the GO editorial team did not agree with a missing *is-a* relation between "*histone methylation*" (GO:0016571) and "*peptidyl-lysine methylation*" (GO:0018022). The first layer of evidence leveraged by our approach to suggest this relation is an existing *is-a* relation between "*histone acetylation*" (GO:0016573) and "*peptidyl-lysine acetylation*" (GO:0018394). According to the GO editorial team, histones can also be methylated on residues other than lysine, while it looks like that acetylation is only on lysines [137].

Limitations

When generating lexical patterns for concept pairs, we require that the two concepts in a concept pair need to share at least one common word. Therefore, the suggested missing relations are among such concept pairs with common words. Since over 99% of concepts in GO have at least one unrelated concept with common words, almost all the GO concepts were considered for missing relation identification by this approach. However, there might be other missing relations among concept pairs that do not share any common words that this approach misses. In the future, we plan to explore whether leveraging ancestors' lexical features could help identify relational defects for concept pairs without common words.

In addition, certain lexical patterns generated by our approach may be similar and could be further grouped or generalized. For instance, the following two lexical patterns (see Table 6.7) are similar:

$$([K_1, K_2, K_3, K_4, \text{"}differentiation\text{"}], [K_1, K_2, K_3, K_4, \text{"}activation\text{"}]);$$

$$and ([K_1, \text{"}differentiation\text{"}], [K_1, \text{"}activation\text{"}]).$$

These two lexical patterns could be grouped and generalized to a single lexical pattern:

$$([K, \text{"}differentiation\text{"}], [K, \text{"}activation\text{"}]),$$

where K represents one or more common words between the two concepts. Such generalization may uncover additional potentially missing relations as the pattern does not require a specific number of common words.

Since a lexical pattern can be generated by a pair of concepts with an indirect relation (through reasoning rules in Table 6.6), an identified missing relation using this lexical pattern may also be indirect. That is, there may be an intermediate missing relation (which is more specific) from which the former missing relation can be inferred. Given the significant amount of manual effort needed to uncover such intermediate missing relations, it is highly desirable to develop automated or semi-automated methods that can identify such root cause issues that lead to the indirect missing relations.

Although our approach is capable of automatically suggesting potentially missing relations based on two layers of evidence, the manual evaluation by domain experts showed that a few cases revealed erroneous existing relations. It remains a challenge to automatically identify such erroneous existing relations to further reduce manual effort by domain experts.

Conclusion: In this section, we presented an evidence-based approach to identify relational defects regarding *is-a*, *part-of*, *has-part*, *regulates*, *negatively regulates*, and *positively regulates* relationships in GO. We were able to automatically extract lexical patterns from concept pairs and difference patterns from concept quadruples as two layers of evidence to suggest potentially missing relations. Both local domain experts' evaluation and GO consortium's encouraging feedback indicated the effectiveness of our evidence-based approach, which can be utilized to uncover missing relations and erroneous existing relations in GO.

Visualization and Retrospective Ground-Truthing 7

7.1 Retrieving and Rendering Non-lattice Substructures

Visualization of SNOMED CT's non-lattice subgraphs can help make sense of what has been asserted in the hierarchical (*is-a*) relation. More importantly, it can demonstrate what has not been asserted, or "is-not-a," using Closed-World Assumption for such subgraphs. Existing browsers such as the SNOMED CT Browser [138] and the NLM SNOMED CT Browser [139] were not designed to support the interactive visualization of non-lattice subgraphs. The size and complexity of SNOMED CT require sophisticated techniques to handle algorithmic, perceptual, and real-time visualization challenges [140]. Hundreds of thousands of non-lattice pairs and non-lattice subgraphs exist in each version of SNOMED CT, making speedy construction of such subgraphs a difficult task. For example, 631,006 non-lattice pairs and 171,011 non-lattice, non-comparable subgraphs were found in the September 2015 version of SNOMED CT (US edition). An efficient searching interface is also indispensable to quickly locate non-lattice subgraphs of interest after they have been generated. Since lattice and non-lattice structures are specific types of directed acyclic graphs (DAGs), classical graph rendering algorithms, and techniques need to be adapted and implemented for visualizing subgraphs in ontological systems.

To overcome such challenges, we introduce a visualization tool called Web-based Interactive Visualization of Non-Lattice Subgraphs (WINS). WINS can effectively display all relevant information around non-lattice subgraphs specified by a user in virtually real-time while allowing the user to perform meaningful interaction with the ontological substructure. This section serves as a use case for WINS dedicated to supporting non-lattice subgraph visualization for facilitating quality assurance of SNOMED CT.

© The Author(s), under exclusive license to Springer Nature Switzerland AG 2022
G.-Q. Zhang et al., *Formal Methods for the Analysis of Biomedical Ontologies*,
Synthesis Lectures on Data, Semantics, and Knowledge,
https://doi.org/10.1007/978-3-031-12131-9_7

7.1.1   Conjunctive Navigational Exploration

Searching is the process that helps people locate relevant information from an existing collection. Typically, a user provides a textual query, and the search engine presents a ranked document list in accordance with the computed degree of relevance. However, such searching process is not always effective in supporting navigation and browsing while also locating the targeted results. *Lookup* and *exploratory* are two basic search modes in information retrieval. In the lookup mode, a user knows precisely what to look for, enters search terms, and tries to get the corresponding set of responses. While in the exploratory mode, a user may not be able to easily and effectively formulate a descriptive search term, and must rely on navigational mechanisms such as menus or facets [141] to browse and explore the content. A single search mode may not handle all searching requirements, especially when the volume of search results can be overwhelmingly large and needs to be further structured to allow relevant information to be located. Conjunctive exploratory navigation interfaces CENI and SCENI [142–144] have been developed for exploring consumer health questions with health topics as dynamically search tags complementing keyword-based lookup. The conjunctive exploration mechanism allows users to quickly narrow down to the most relevant results in the most effective way.

7.1.2   Components of WINS

WINS follows a Model-View-Controller (MVC) design principle. Figure 7.1 illustrates the system architecture of WINS. WINS uses MongoDB as the backend database to store non-lattice subgraphs extracted from SNOMED CT. The view mainly contains four parts: (a) facet options; (b) query widgets; (c) result display panel; and (d) graph rendering. Controller connects the model and view. Query translator converts user's search requests to mongoDB queries. The query results are then sent to topological sort and position calculation algorithms to obtain formatted data for D3.js to render non-lattice subgraphs.

Generating Non-lattice Subgraphs

As discussed in Sect. 4.1, non-lattice fragments are graphs consisting of the concepts between any member of the non-lattice pair and any member of their maximal lower bounds.

However, it is possible that multiple non-lattice pairs have identical maximal lower bounds. In this case, multiple non-lattice fragments will share the same maximal lower bounds, which could involve redundant work in analyzing each of these fragments. To avoid such redundant work, the definition of "non-lattice subgraph" has been introduced in Sect. 5.2. A non-lattice subgraph is determined by a non-lattice pair and its maximal lower bounds. We generate non-lattice subgraphs for WINS by only including the minimal concepts sharing the same maximal lower bounds. Given a non-lattice pair p and its maximal

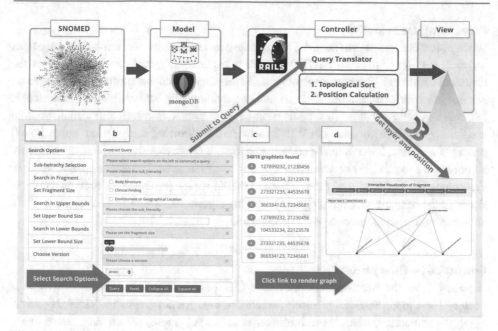

Fig. 7.1 Functional architecture: **a**. facet options; **b**. query widgets; **c**. query results; **d**. graph rendering

Fig. 7.2 An example of non-lattice subgraph of size 6. Nodes represent concepts and edges represent *is-a* relations

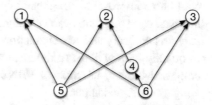

lower bounds $mlb(p)$, a non-lattice subgraph can be obtained by (1) reversely computing the minimal upper bounds of the maximal lower bounds, denoted by $mub(mlb(p))$, and (2) aggregating all the concepts and edges between (including) any concept in $mub(mlb(p))$ and any of the maximal lower bounds $mlb(p)$. We call $mub(mlb(p))$ and $mlb(p)$ the upper bounds and lower bounds of the non-lattice subgraph, respectively. The size of a non-lattice subgraph is defined as the number of concepts it contains. For instance, given a non-lattice pair (1, 2) and its maximal lower bounds {5, 6} as shown in Fig. 7.2, computing the minimal upper bounds of {5, 6} yields {1, 2, 3}. Then the non-lattice subgraph contains all the concepts and relations between {1, 2, 3} and {5, 6}, that is, concepts {1, 2, 3, 4, 5, 6} and *is-a* relations {(5, 1), (5, 2), (5, 3), (6, 1), (6, 4), (4, 2), (6, 3)}. In this case, we aggregate three non-lattice fragments {1, 2, 4, 5, 6}, {1, 3, 5, 6}, and {2, 3, 4, 5, 6} into one non-lattice subgraph.

Processing Data Model

We followed the approach in Sect. 4.3 to compute non-lattice pairs and non-lattice subgraphs for each version of SNOMED CT. We store non-lattice subgraphs in MongoDB in the format of document. The advantage of using MongoDB and document format is that we do not need to restrict to specific schemas and can dynamically extend existing data models with customized attributes. To support facet-based conjunctive search and visualization, a non-lattice subgraph document in WINS includes the following information: upper bound concepts and size, lower bound concepts and size, total size of the non-lattice subgraph, all concepts and relations between them, synonyms, hierarchical information, and version. Pre-computed upper and lower closures as a table of triples $(c, \uparrow c, \downarrow c)$ for each concept c is stored in the database to speed up graph rendering algorithms, where $\uparrow c$ denotes concept c's ancestors and $\downarrow c$ denotes concept c's descendants.

Conjunctive Query Interface

Benefited from the mechanism developed in CENI [142, 143], a novel search method is designed to support fast and precisely locating non-lattice subgraphs in WINS. By leveraging the semantic and structural information in the subgraphs, we create a set of query facets to help narrow down the search scope, such as the subgraph size. Another feature is that words and metadata are extracted and serve as topic tags for each subgraph, which could help improve the relevance of search results. This search method allows the user to navigate to specific non-lattice subgraphs in multiple ways. The WINS search interface supports arbitrary logical conjunction of options and provides the user with multiple paths to quickly narrow down to the most relevant contents. Figure 7.3 shows the layout of the conjunctive query interface of WINS. It contains the query options panel and the query widgets construction panel.

Query facets allow users to navigate through different topics of the search results. In WINS, we have 9 facet options (shown in Fig. 7.3): search terms in upper bounds and lower bounds of subgraphs; search terms in concept descriptions of subgraphs; search by the subgraph size, upper bound size, or lower bound size; search in a specific hierarchy; search in a specific SNOMED CT version, and search a pair of concepts. By selecting one option at a time, in an incremental fashion, a user arrives at narrower and narrower content areas that are relevant to all the options selected so far, conjunctively. For example, searching "chronic heart disease" in the concept descriptions of subgraphs obtains 214 non-lattice subgraphs; and further setting the subgraph size as a range of 4 to 6 obtains 15 non-lattice subgraphs.

Each time a facet is selected, the corresponding query widget will pop up in the query construction panel. The user can enter specific search requirements in each of these query widgets. WINS has several types of widgets to make the inputting easier. Text box is used for entering strings; slider bar is used for setting size; drop-down menu is used for selecting versions; and radio button is used for choosing hierarchies. As shown in Fig. 7.3, users can remove one widget by clicking its "X" or remove all selected widgets by clicking the "Reset"

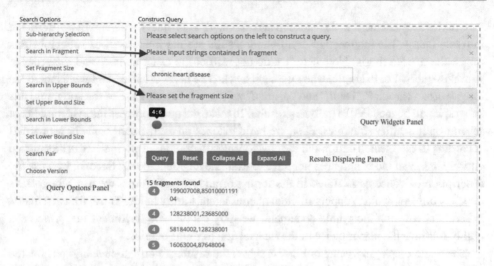

Fig. 7.3 Conjunctive query interface of WINS

button. "Collapse All" and "Expand All" are used when the list of query widgets is too long. By clicking "Query" button, all the query constraints in this area will be translated into MongoDB queries through the controller of WINS.

Algorithm 1: Topological sort for layers.

1 **Function** *Topological Sort(C)*
        Data: Upper bounds u, nodes $N, adj[][]$
        Result: $layer[]$
2   index $i = 1$
3        $layer[u] = i$
4        $visited[u] = u$
5   queue q.push(u)
6   **while** *q not empty* **do**
7            $u' = q$.pop()
8            $i = i + 1$
9   **foreach** $n \in N$ **do**
10   **if** $adj[u'][n]$ *is true and* $visited[n]$ *is false* **then**
11                   $layer[n] = i$ and $visited[n] = true$
12   q.push(n)
13   **end**
14   **end**
15   **end**
16 **return** $layer[]$

Queries are generated in the backend and executed. Each query widget will be translated into one query. The intersection of all query results are the final result of subgraphs that match the query criteria. Note here, we do not restrict the exact number and the order of words in query. For example, when we search "chronic heart disease," as long as there are three words "chronic," "heart," and "disease" existing in one concept of the subgraph, this subgraph will be included in the query results. To make the query process fast, we implement several optimization strategies. First, we build indexes on all the subgraphs in MongoDB according to each search option and use covered query technique, a query that can be satisfied entirely using an index and does not have to examine any documents. Second, because the description of concepts is stored in the format of an array of words, we use MongoDB's *multikey indexes*, which support efficient queries against array fields. Third, for each query, instead of returning the whole document, we only capture the document ids, which can highly improve the performance of the intersection of multi-queries.

The result displaying panel in Fig. 7.3 shows the result of non-lattice subgraphs related to the constructed query, displayed in the ascending order of subgraph sizes. The number in the green circle denotes the size of the subgraph, and is followed by a hyper-link showing the identifiers of upper bound concepts of the subgraph. When clicking on these identifiers, the subgraph will be rendered in a new page in the browser.

Interactive Visualization

Visualization in WINS is created using force-layout form of D3.js, one of the most popular dynamic and interactive data visualization libraries. Since ontology and non-lattice subgraphs are directed acyclic graph, hierarchical (top-down) layouts are easy for users to understand. We use Algorithm 1 (*topological sort*) to assign each node in a subgraph a layer number. When rendering the non-lattice subgraph, nodes in the same layer are drawn at the same vertical level. Several heuristic features have been put forth to capture the visual aesthetics of a graph, including minimizing the number of edge crossings, coloring different types of nodes, minimizing overlapping of text, and maintaining symmetry.

Figure 7.4 shows the graph rendering page for non-lattice subgraphs. The green nodes represent the upper bounds of the subgraph, the purple ones represent lower bounds, and the gray lines represent *is-a* relations. WINS also provides additional features to make this visualization tool functional and interactive. Users can choose to show the parents of the upper bounds and the children of lower bounds of the subgraph and highlight primitive concepts and stated relations to make them different from defined and inferred ones, which are useful functions for investigating the subgraph. Since the graph is Scalable Vector Graphics (SVG) rendered by D3.js, users can drag the nodes and edges to make the subgraph easy to read, especially for large ones. If a user believes the subgraph is interesting, he or she can save the subgraph for further investigation and also can share the finding to others, by clicking "Save Subgraph" and "Share Subgraph" button respectively. Besides, user can download

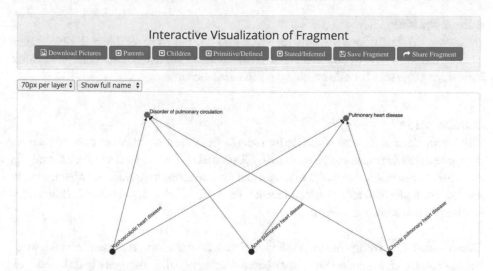

Fig. 7.4 Subgraph rendering page of WINS

the graph in various formats including SVG, PNG, and TIKZ. Subgraph editing function is also available in WINS.

7.1.3 Performance Evaluation of the Layout Algorithm

We used the distribution files of SNOMED CT (US edition) to generate non-lattice subgraphs. From the March 2012 version to the September 2018 version, we have generated 14 versions of non-lattice subgraphs and stored them into the database, along with the corresponding concepts, relations, and term dictionaries.

The time complexity of the layout algorithm needs to be low to maintain efficient interaction with users. From our experiments, It was seen that, even for size of 40, it only takes about 4ms, which indicates a reasonable rendering time. For detailed results, analysis, and discussions about the findings of this work, please see [145].

7.1.4 Strengths and Limitations of WINS

Interactive Visualization

Although WINS provides a practical and efficient method for users to access and visualize non-lattice subgraphs, there are limitations as well. It highly relies on domain experts to manually check each subgraph and provide remediation suggestions. One possible solution is to use Formal Concept Analysis to automatically suggest missing concepts and relations for each subgraph. Other lexical or structural auditing methods can also be good supplements to enhance WINS to support automatic or semi-automatic ontology quality assurance work.

Generalizability

WINS was originally designed only for SNOMED CT, but its general and flexible system architecture allows it to be able to serve as a framework for similar systems that can visualize non-lattice subgraphs for other ontologies such as Gene Ontology.

Collaboration

WINS provides a community function for users to share the assessment of their findings, so change recommendations can be accessed by SNOMED CT editorial committee directly. In the "share" page, users can post a subgraph and the correction suggestions. Other users can join the discussion and make their comments. Voting function is also included. Basically, it functions like a common forum.

Conclusions: This section presents WINS, an interactive platform for visualizing the structures of ontologies to support non-lattice based ontology quality assurance and shared decision making. The purpose of WINS is to provide a browser for users to access, retrieve, and visualize non-lattice subgraphs in identifying the most promising areas for quality assurance. WINS is designed to serve as a community portal for SNOMED CT developers and users to perform collaborative graph-sensemaking and change recommendation. Our preliminary results suggest that WINS has fulfilled these design objectives.

7.2   Leveraging Evolutionary Changes

Finding errors in existing ontologies is a creative discovery process. Because of the highly discovery-oriented nature of Ontology Quality Assurance (OQA), the performance measure of *precision* (i.e., the percentage of true errors among the candidates that have been examined) for auditing methods is neither an initial consideration nor as glorious to quantify, unlike the setting for information retrieval [146]. Similarly, *recall*, the percentage of errors discovered among *all true errors* ("the ground truth"), is impossible to measure because of the lack of ground truth: a complete, validated error list is impossible to construct, again because of the highly discovery-oriented nature of the task.

Nevertheless, reference standards, or benchmarking data sets with validated results, have played critical roles for advancing disciplines such as image analysis (e.g., Face Recognition Technology [147] and Wilt Dataset [148]) and information retrieval (e.g., The Text Retrieval Conference series (http://trec.nist.gov)), and would be an important resource for OQA. Despite the fact that it is impossible to obtain precision and recall measures for OQA methods in absolute terms, it may still be meaningful to investigate such measures relative to some "partial ground truth."

Our goals here are twofold: to develop reference sets for evaluating the performance of OQA methods for SNOMED CT, and to demonstrate how such reference sets may be applied to evaluate the performance of lattice versus non-lattice-based methods with randomized review as a background benchmark. We propose RGT, Retrospective Ground-Truthing, as a surrogate reference standard for evaluating the performance of automated OQA methods. The key idea of RGT is to leverage the cumulative SNOMED CT changes derived from its regular longitudinal distributions by the official SNOMED CT editorial board as a partial, surrogate reference standard. Three performance measure are proposed: *RGT recall*, *RGT precision*, and *RGT geometric mean (G-measure)*, formulated by adapting the standard measures using RGT relational changes derived from SNOMED CT U.S. distributions as the reference set.

7.2.1   Obtaining and Using Retrospective Ground-Truthing

We first construct a partial reference set focusing on two types of relational errors derived from the "delta" of SNOMED CT releases: incorrect *is-a* relations represented by *is-a* deletions, and missing *is-a* relations as captured by *is-a* insertions. We then perform a comparative evaluation of lattice, non-lattice, and randomized relational auditing methods using the standard precision, recall, and geometric measures.

Constructing Retrospective Ground-Truthing

We use 5 versions (U.S. version 20140301—U.S. version 20160901) of SNOMED CT for capturing relational changes. We focus on erroneous and missing relations on shared concepts, so newly added relations that involve newly added concepts are ignored. An *is-a* relational change (or *is-a* change in short) with the same source and target concepts may have different "modualId," which may cause a repeated count. Moreover, *is-a* relations may be reversed back to a prior version as a part of the changes in later versions [41]. For example, relation "*Streptococcal tonsillitis*" (41582007) *is-a* "*Tonsillitis*" (90176007) is deleted in the July 2014 version and added in the January 2016 version. To construct a robust reference set of relational changes, we perform three preprocessing steps:

- Extracting only *is-a* changes;
- Removing duplicated counts and reversed changes; and
- Removing *is-a* changes that involve concepts not in the targeted SNOMED CT versions.

Extracting Independent Lattice and Non-lattice Fragments

We first extract all lattice and non-lattice fragments for the U.S. version 20140301 of SNOMED CT using the MapReduce pipeline discussed in Sect. 4.2, which consists two MapReduce phases to extract non-lattice fragments from large partially ordered ontological structures. The resulting fragments are not "independent" in the sense that one fragment

Fig. 7.5 An example of a
non-lattice fragment containing
a subfragment

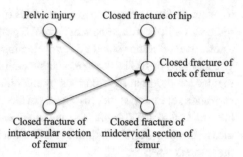

may be contained in another, making further error detection intertwined, as well as violating the independent sampling assumption for statistical analysis. However, given a large collection of fragments, obtaining a reduced "independent" collection with exhaustive pairwise comparison is computationally prohibitive. To address this issue, we formulate the notion of *independence* as follows. For (induced and connected) fragments $f_1 = (C_1, R_1)$ and $f_2 = (C_2, R_2)$ where C_1 and C_2 are sets of concepts and R_1 and R_2 are sets of relations,

- we say that f_2 is a subfragment of f_1 if $R_2 \subseteq R_1$; and
- we say that f_1 and f_2 are independent f neither of them is a subgragment of the other.

For example, the non-lattice fragment in Fig. 7.5 shows the non-lattice fragment generated by the non-lattice pair "*Pelvic injury*" (282771003) and "*Closed fracture of hip*" (359817006) has a non-lattice subfragment generated by the non-lattice pair "*Pelvic injury*" (282771003) and "*Closed fracture of neck of femur*" (35982003).

In general, a collection of fragments is called *independent* if each pair of fragments from the collection is independent.

Formally, for a non-lattice pair (a, b) and their maximal lower bounds $\mathrm{mlb}\{a, b\}$, the *non-lattice fragment* determined by the pair (a, b) is defined as a subgraph containing the concepts between the pair (a, b) and any concept in $\mathrm{mlb}\{a, b\}$. For a lattice pair (c, d), their only maximal lower bound is the unique element in $\mathrm{mlb}\{c, d\}$, and their only minimun upper bound is the unique element in $\mathrm{mub}\{c, d\}$, the *lattice fragment* determined by the pair (c, d) is defined as a subgraph containing the concepts between the pair (c, d) and the concept $\mathrm{mlb}\{c, d\}$, combining the concepts between the pair (a, b) and the concept $\mathrm{mub}\{a, b\}$. The MapReduce pipeline in Sect. 4.2 can be used to exhaustively detect non-lattice and lattice pairs. We further compute independent fragments using the generating pairs.

By definition, comparing all relations between every pair of fragments is required for constructing an dependent collection of non-lattice fragments. To reduce the computational cost involved, we propose an algorithm to detect all possible non-lattice subfragments for each given non-lattice fragment. Lattice fragment dependency can be computed in a similar way.

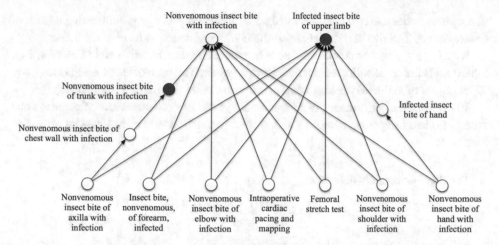

Fig. 7.6 An example of an independent non-lattice fragment containing a non-lattice pair (colored in red) other than that pair generated the fragment. The non-lattice fragment generated by the pair in red is not contained in the displayed fragment

Let P be the set of all non-lattice pairs, and F be the set of all non-lattice fragments for a given SNOMED CT version. Every non-lattice fragment $f_{(a,b)} \in F$ is generated by some non-lattice pair $(a, b) \in P$. Then $f_{(x,y)}$ is subfragment of $f_{(a,b)}$ if

- $(x, y) \neq (a, b)$, $(x, y) \in P$, $\{x, y\} \subseteq f_{(a,b)}$; and
- for any relation $(u, v) \in f_{(x,y)}$, we have $(u, v) \in f_{(a,b)}$.

The second condition is required because a non-lattice pair may generate a non-lattice fragment without itself being a part of the fragment. For instance, the non-lattice fragment in Fig. 7.6 shows an independent non-lattice fragment generated by the non-lattice pair "*Nonvenomous insect bite with infection*" (10461000) and "*Infected insect bite of upper limb*" (283347003). This fragment contains another non-lattice pair "*Nonvenomous insect bite of trunk with infection*" (19108007) and "*Infected insect bite of upper limb*" (283347003), although this pair does not generate a subfragment of the displayed fragment.

Performance Measures

To the best of our knowledge, there are no existing measures to compare distinct OQA methods. We introduce *RGT recall*, *RGT precision*, and *RGT geometric mean* to measure the performance of OQA methods, motivated by the precision and recall measures commonly used in information retrieval.

We consider an OQA method M as a group of fragments (in general terms as induced subgraphs). Each fragment may potentially capture some ontological errors that involve concepts as nodes and *is-a* relations as edges. A fragment f is a graph consisting of a set of *is-a* relations. The size of f is defined as the number of concepts involved in it.

We can view a benchmark of validated changes (i.e., ground truth) a tuple $\mathcal{E} = (E_0, E_1)$, where E_0 is the set of validated relational errors (where a relation deletion is indicated), and E_1 is the set of validated missing relations (where a relation insertion is indicated).

To evaluate the performance of M against $\mathcal{E}$, we can break the measure of precision and recall into two categories: measures with respect to deletion, and measures with respect to insertion:

- The deletion recall is defined as

$$\frac{|\{r \in E_0 \mid \exists f \in M, r \in f\}|}{|E_0|};$$

- The deletion precision is defined as

$$\frac{|\{f \in M \mid \exists r \in f, r \in E_0\}|}{|M|};$$

- The insertion recall is defined as

$$\frac{|\{r \in E_1 \mid \exists f \in M, r \in f\}|}{|E_1|};$$

- The insertion precision is defined as

$$\frac{|\{f \in M \mid \exists r \in f, r \in E_1\}|}{|M|}.$$

One can combine precision and recall to obtain the geometric mean measure (G-measure) $\sqrt{\text{recall} \cdot \text{precision}}$. The G-measure shows a combined performance of precision and recall. The higher the G-measure, the greater the agreement between an OQA method and the SNOMED CT changes.

7.2.2   Findings in SNOMED CT

Relational changes in SNOMED CT U.S. versions ranged from 19,753 in the 20160901 release to 64,676 in the 20160301 release. All the changes were calculated based on the released "delta" set for each version. There has been a total of cumulative 263,994 relational changes from the 20140301 release to the 20160901 release, after removing relation reversals and duplicates. Therefore, the cumulative change is not a simple summation of the numbers in all prior changes.

We compared five auditing methods according to our formulation of each method as a collection of fragments. Non-lattice auditing consists of all non-lattice fragments and

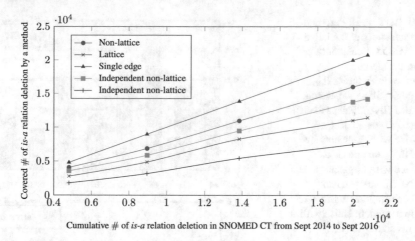

Fig. 7.7 Number of incorrect *is-a* relationships discovered by method over cumulative *is-a* relationship deletion in SNOMED CT

lattice auditing consists of all lattice fragments. Similarly, independent non-lattice auditing consists of all independent non-lattice fragments and independent lattice auditing consists of all independent lattice fragments. Additionally, single-edge auditing consists of all fragments made of a single relation (edge). This corresponds to randomized edge examination.

We used March 2014 version of SNOMED CT to generate non-lattice fragments, lattice fragments, and single-edge fragments. From lattice and non-lattice fragments, we extracted all independent fragments and divided them into large size group and small size group.

For RGT recall in detecting incorrect *is-a* relationship errors, we found that the measure for each method is almost a constant. Figure 7.7 shows the number of SNOMED CT *is-a* relationship deletion discovered through method over the number of 5 versions SNOMED CT *is-a* relationship deletion accumulation (4,799; 8,965; 13,844; 19,968; and 20,744) from version September 2014 to version September 2016. For each of five method groups, the slope is the RGT recall, and the larger the slope is, the better RGT recall the method has. The line of best fitting for each method is linear which indicates that the RGT recall is stable with different SNOMED CT *is-a* relationship deletion numbers for all methods. Such feature proves that RGT recall is a good measure for OQA method evaluation. And with such feature, we can predict that the incorrect *is-a* relationship errors detection recall relative to the ground truth for a method is very close to its RGT recall relative to SNOMED CT *is-a* relationship deletion.

Figure 7.8 displays the results of RGT recall and RGT precision on detecting incorrect *is-a* relationship errors for each method. Figure 7.9 displays the results of RGT recall and RGT precision on detecting missing *is-a* relationship errors for each method. Table 7.1 displays the results of the G-measure of RGT recall and RGT precision on detecting incorrect *is-a*

Fig. 7.8 RGT recall (left) and
RGT precision (right) relative
to SNOMED CT relationship
deletion for methods
non-lattice (NL), lattice (L),
single-edge (SE), independent
non-lattice (INL), independent
lattice (IL), independent
non-lattice with fragments size
≤15 (INLS), independent
non-lattice with fragments size
>15 (INLL), independent
lattice with fragments size ≤15
(ILS), independent lattice with
fragments size >15 (ILL)

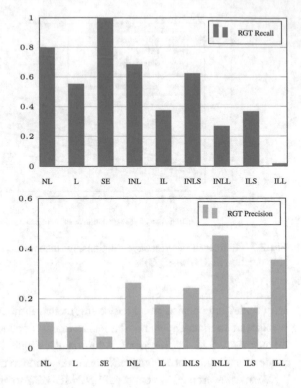

relationship (SNOMED CT *is-a* relationship deletion), missing *is-a* relationship (SNOMED CT *is-a* relationship insertion), and either of the errors for each method.

The first three rows of Table 7.1 show that non-lattice performs better than lattice and much better than single-edge using G-measure. From Figs. 7.8 and 7.9, we found the reason that non-lattice has a higher G-measure is non-lattice has higher RGT recall (79.9% and 53.4%) than lattice while they perform similarly in RGT precision, which means non-lattice has better coverage on incorrect *is-a* relationship errors and missing *is-a* relationship errors. Such result proves that non-lattice structure has more possibility on *is-a* relationship error detection than lattice structure.

Among all methods, independent non-lattice is the best on discovering incorrect *is-a* relationships with a 68.4% RGT recall and a 26.2% RGT precision, which shows that the independent non-lattice fragments play big roles on detecting incorrect *is-a* relationship in the whole ontology graph. Only 68,849 independent non-lattice fragments (about 11% of all non-lattice fragments) exist in SNOMED CT version March 2014, and 62,001 (90%) of them are in small sizes (≤15) so that they are amendable for human inspection. However, independent non-lattice fails to show good performance on discovering missing *is-a* relationships, and non-lattice auditing returns the best G-measure in missing *is-a* relationships detection. The reason is that a missing relationship is often needed to connect a concept inside a non-lattice fragment and another concept outside the non-lattice fragment, then

Fig. 7.9 RGT recall (left) and RGT precision (right) relative to insertion changes for methods non-lattice (NL), lattice (L), single-edge (SE), independent non-lattice (INL), independent lattice (IL), independent non-lattice with fragments size ≤15 (INLS), independent non-lattice with fragments size >15 (INLL), independent lattice with fragments size ≤15 (ILS), independent lattice with fragments size >15 (ILL)

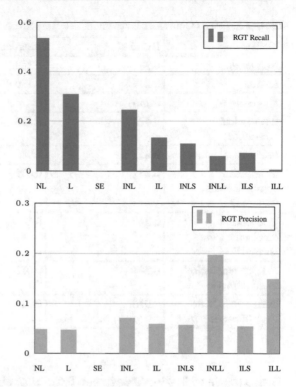

larger non-lattice fragments with dependency are able to catch such missing relationships. The scenario also leads bad insertion discovering result for independent non-lattice because missing relationships are only detected between concepts inside a fragment.

Please see [149] for further details about the findings of this work.

7.2.3 Further Analysis of the Approach

Small G-Scores

Compared with traditional information retrieval methods, the G-scores calculated here are relatively low, even for the higher-performing non-lattice approaches. This should not be a concern for two reasons. One is that SNOMED CT change is continuing with each new release, and we are always dealing with partial ground truth. In lack of the existence of available complete ground truth set, the performances for any OQA methods would suffer. The second reason is that detecting ontology errors or defects is a highly discovery-oriented, and sometimes not even well-defined process. For the first time, this section introduced a framework to provide the feasibility to calculate G-scores to enable the comparison of distinct OQA methods (but the comparative evaluation of some existing OQA methods may remain infeasible).

Table 7.1 List of G-measure for methods detecting SNOMED CT changes

Method	Deletion	Insertion	Both
Non-lattice	0.291	**0.160**	0.288
Lattice	0.215	0.120	0.215
Single-edge	0.216	0	0.173
Independent non-lattice	**0.423**	0.132	**0.373**
Independent lattice	0.255	0.089	0.226
Independent non-lattice small (size≤15)	0.387	0.079	0.298
Independent non-lattice large (size>15)	0.348	0.107	0.273
Independent lattice small (size≤15)	0.244	0.062	0.190
Independent lattice large (size>15)	0.076	0.026	0.061

Comparison of Methods Between Fragment Sizes

By comparing methods with larger fragments sizes and smaller fragments sizes, methods with larger fragments always show better RGT precision than the methods with smaller fragments. It is intuitive that larger fragments have more concepts and relationships so that they have more possibility to contain errors. On the contrary, methods with smaller size fragments present better scores on RGT recall relative to deletion and insertion, which means SNOMED CT *is-a* relationship changes are aggregated on small sizes of fragments.

Comparison of Populations Between Methods

Independent non-lattice auditing performed best among the three evaluated methods, with merely 68, 849 fragments. To demonstrate the statistical significance, we computed test statistic Z-scores on precision between non-lattice and lattice (35.5); independent non-lattice and independent lattice (46.8); independent non-lattice and single-edge (201.2); and independent lattice and single-edge (149.3). Independent non-lattice auditing departs the most in outcome from larger population sets consisting of individual *is-a* relations.

Balance of RGT Precision and Recall

Our setup for ontology auditing methods to capture quality issues is analogus to capturing fishes using fishing nets. A single method provides a collection of fishing nets. The fishes are the cumulative changes approved by the SNOMED CT editoral panel that have been officially reflected the releases. The nets are the SNOMED CT subsets or fragments determined by a particular method. To illustrate the possibility in the extremes, a method may provide a single net, which is the entire graph of SNOMED CT (100% recall, 100% precision against RGT reference set). But this is useless since no progress is made in making "the haystack" smaller. Another method may provide the finest possible net, which consists of single *is-a* relations. This is also useless since it is equivalent to random examination, because of the largest possible numbers of "fishing nets" used. A more useful method should balance the number of "nets" as well as the sizes of the "nets." We believe this is achieved using independent non-lattice fragments with sizes not exceeding 15.

SNOMED CT Changes Versus the Ground Truth of Relational Errors

The entirety of the ground truth of ontology errors is unknowable because the lack of a complete and validated error list is the inherent nature of the task for OQA. SNOMED CT changes is the most trustworthy error list since it has been generated by the world's most authoritive group - the SNOMED International Editorial Panel. However, there exist change reversals [41] that need to be accounted for, as is the case in this study.

Limitations of Non-lattice Auditing

As discussed in Sect. 4.1, non-lattice auditing is founded on the theory of formal concept analysis. This section demonstrates a significant difference between the G-scores of lattice vs non-lattice based methods in their ability in capturing official SNOMED CT relational changes. However, knowing a non-lattice fragment contains a relational error and identifying this specific error remains two different matters, as each fragment still contains multiple relations. To address this issue, we developed data mining techniques discussed in Sect. 5.2 leverging structural and lexical information for automated detection of relational errors in non-lattice fragments. Further development of data mining techniqies combining a rich variety of information sources represent provide additional research opportunities in this area.

Changes in the Number of Non-lattice Fragments Between Versions

The number of non-lattice fragments can be a significant measure to evaluate the quality of SNOMED CT. We computed the numbers of non-lattice fragments for 4 pairs of versions using shared common concepts between versions: 581,327 (version 20140301) and 575,927 (version 20140901), 562,819 (version 20140901) and 574,028 (version 20150301), 596,015 (version 20150301) and 587,263 (version 20150901), 610,785 (version 20150901) and 604,221 (version 20160301). We did not include the latest version in the comparison because of the sudden drop in the number of relational changes. 3 of 4 pairs showed a decrease of the number of non-lattice fragments. This may suggest that quality assurance work between these versions actually reduced the number of non-lattice fragments. However, the reasons for the unexpected increase in the 20150301 release may need further investigation.

SNOMED CT Versions Used for RGT

We used the latest five versions of SNOMED CT (the March 2017 version was released too late to be included in this study) for feasibility demonstration of our method. This choice was purely a matter of convenience and did not result from methodological or computational limitations of our approach. In fact, it would be desirable to use all the available SNOMED CT versions (in Release Format 1 as well as Release Format 2), with an appropriate starting release as the time-point for computing the fragments. One might only want to go so far to reach a point of relatively stable version (with the sizes of delta sets within a reasonable range). All the performance measures would only improve as the RGT reference set will become larger. We also noted an abnormality in the sudden drop of relational changes in the 20160901 release, which needs further investigation.

Conclusion: This section introduced an innovative notion of RGT reference set for SNOMED CT relational changes and performed a comparative evaluation of the performances of lattice, non-lattice, and randomized relational error detection methods using the standard precision, recall, and geometric measures. An RGT relational-change reference set of $32, 241$ *is-a* changes were constructed from 5 versions of SNOMED CT from September 2014 to September 2016, with reversals and changes due to deletion or addition of new concepts excluded. $68, 849$ independent non-lattice fragments, $118, 587$ independent lattice fragments, and $446, 603$ relations were extracted from the SNOMED CT March 2014 distribution. Comparative performance analysis of smaller (less than 15) lattice versus non-lattice fragments were also given to reflect the more realistic setting in which such methods may be applied. Among the $32, 241$ *is-a* changes, independent non-lattice fragments covered 52.8% changes with 26.4% precision with a G-score of 0.373, showing non-lattice auditing as a more superior approach than using lattices, confirming a theoretical predication implicitly given in Sect. 4.1.

Conclusion

8

The six main content chapters of the book provided approaches for analyzing ontological structure and content with the goal of detecting potential quality issues (errors, inconsistencies, or gaps in concept entities as well as their relations) and enhancing quality of the knowledge represented. Central to our approach has been the theory of Formal Concept Analysis (Sect. 1.2.3) as a general mathematical underpinning for lattice-conformation of the *is-a* relation as an ontological principle (Sect. 1.2.2).

8.1   Formal Concept Analysis and the Lattice-Conformation Principle

Formal Concept Analysis has been a mathematical framework for studying abstract thinking. Abstract concepts serve as the fundamental blocks of human cognition, as exemplified by biomedical ontologies covered in this book. In FCA, a concept is treated as a pair of its extent (objects) and its intent (attributes), and the duality between the two is characterized by a precisely defined mathematical structure called a Galois connection. For example, if one translates an English passage to Russian, and then translate the resulting Russian passage back to English *while preserving the original meaning*, then a Galois connection is established.

This book exploited FCA in a couple of ways.

One was at the overall structural level, based on the fundamental theorem of FCA: the order structure of formal concepts is always a complete lattice. Given this, if we see an ontological hierarchy (i.e., *is-a*) relation not to be a complete lattice or lattice, then we have a problem: a situation violating the mathematical theory of FCA. This meta-level reasoning or dialog was captured in Figs. 1.7 and 1.8. In order to apply this lattice-conformation principle to ontological structures, we needed to be able to automatically find or detect substructures that violate the lattice property. This required the development of efficient

G.-Q. Zhang et al., *Formal Methods for the Analysis of Biomedical Ontologies*,
Synthesis Lectures on Data, Semantics, and Knowledge,
https://doi.org/10.1007/978-3-031-12131-9_8

non-lattice detection algorithms (Sects. 4.1, 4.2), non-lattice fragment extraction procedures (Sect. 4.3), and visualization methods for human sensemaking (Sect. 7.1, and examples in the Appendix). Once non-lattice fragments were extracted, the question became what specific edges in the fragment were potentially problematic. For this step, i.e., *automatically generating recommended changes*, it is inevitable that we needed to use lexical information contained in concept names (labels) to pinpoint the inconsistencies that may have resulted in non-lattice-conforming "behavior" for the fragment. In general, our experience has been that a non-lattice fragment is almost always indicative of certain issues. These issues were sometimes easier to identify and fix *automatically*, and other times highly non-trivial and pointed to core challenges in ontological engineering that source owners and editors were already aware of.

The second was specifically invoking the processes dictated by FCA by constructing an appropriate formal context, constructing the corresponding concept lattice next, and then comparing the resulting structure with the ontological fragment of interest. This has been the focus of Chap. 3. This approach is more complex and computationally more demanding, as it involved the selection of a set of concepts as objects, keywords or relation targets as attributes, and then the algorithm for constructing the corresponding concept lattices for each fragment of interest, as well as the comparison of two ordered structures in each instance for (non)-isomorphism mapping.

The third was the use of properly rendered non-lattice fragments in our manual evaluation of the various methods by domain experts. Without the ability to render and print the identified errors and recommended changes within the originating non-lattice fragments, our evaluations performed by domain experts would have been harder, unintuitive, and more time-consuming. With the exhibited contextual information provided in the non-lattice fragments, the inconsistencies and errors became more pronounced and easier to spot. To illustrate this, we devoted pages in the Appendix to show how small non-lattice fragments already provided sufficient information for correctly recommended changes that were confirmed by domain experts (most of them are expected to have already been incorporated into newer releases of the ontology). Incidentally, as we expected, all the corrected structures became lattice-conforming. Therefore, as errors are corrected, non-lattice structures were eliminated in the process. This also suggests the inverse of the *number of non-lattice fragments in an ontological hierarchy* as a quality metric, although a more systematic investigation of this metric is beyond the scope of this work (some hints for this were given in Sect. 7.2).

8.2   Lexical Sequences and Structural Relations

Independent of formal concept analysis, a lot can be leveraged by closer examination of normalized concept names. Treating them as a "bag of words" can be simple and effective for identifying certain errors (Chap. 2). But treating them authentically as word sequences as they appear in concept names, coupled with associated relations, can be even more powerful (Chap. 6). Lexical subsequence structures (after proper subgrouping and nesting) and associated alignment patterns have the potential to provide more in-depth information about the semantics that a concept class is intended to capture.

8.3   Scalability of Algorithms

As emphasized at the beginning, desirable ontological analysis algorithms that are most effective for auditing and quality enhancement need to be able to identify specific errors (i.e., "bugs"), automatically make change suggestions and provide "explanation" or reasoning for the suggested changes as well. Such algorithms should be applicable to ontological systems in its entirety for exhaustive analysis. Therefore, the speed of the algorithm is an important aspect to consider. In the extreme, if an algorithm associated with a fictional "perfect" algorithm takes longer (e.g. one year) to finish, then it would be useless because the algorithm would not have finished running before the next release cycle. In this book we have presented several strategies, from using off-the-shelf solutions in SPARQL, MapReduce parallel processing, to novel algorithmic ideas that gets to the root of the computational challenge. In implementing an ontological analysis algorithm, one should consider the expected computational complexity, the effort needed in extracting and presenting change recommendations, and the clarity in providing a concrete rationale for the suggested changes to facilitate human validation. Using a computational complexity analogy, the task of finding potential errors falls into the problem space of *NP*, while the task of accepting or rejecting a change suggestion in terms of the provided "evidence" should be as easy as *P*.

8.4   Performance Metric, Precision and Recall

Finding ontological errors (anomalies, inconsistencies, or incompleteness) is like finding needles in a haystack. Traditionally, ontology quality assurance methods have not subjected to performance evaluation examinations as those popularized by machine learning. Machine learning, on the other hand, cannot be compared to the task of "finding needles in a haystack" either.

Therefore, while it is important to perform rigorous performance evaluation of ontological analysis methods, we should not automatically adopt the notations of precision, recall, and F1 score as performance metrics. Even if we adopt some elements of such natural measures, we should avoid comparing the outcome numbers of machine learning evaluations with ontological analysis evaluations. However, in lack of a true "recall," it may still be possible to establish reference standards, or benchmark libraries so that there is a common standard for comparing and evaluating ontological analysis methods. Chapter 7 of the book, "retrospective ground-truthing," is a straightforward, though imperfect, approach using future releases as reference benchmarks. Informal assessment also uses the strategy of relative comparative analysis: did one method find all errors detected by another (earlier) method, and if not, to what extent it did. One potentially unifying opportunity would be to develop benchmark evaluation libraries (per ontology and per task) so that systematic comparison can be performed against a common "standard." This strategy has shown effectiveness in advancing other fields, such as ImageNet for deep learning.

Auto-suggestion – automatically detecting errors and automatically generating suggested changes – is even more desirable and challenging. Theoretically, detection and change-suggestion methods can be developed and evaluated independently, although in most of our reported work here these two aspects are combined together naturally, especially when using Formal Concept Analysis either directly or indirectly. Given the ultimate goal of enhancing the quality of ontologies, auto-suggestion is a highly desirable capability of any method, and the outcomes of their performance evaluation should be commensurate with the level of difficulty of the tasks such methods aimed to tackle.

8.5   Machine Learning Opportunities

Given that biomedical ontologies are intended to encode declarative knowledge, it seems natural to "learn" from this curated and relatively high-quality knowledge source and apply newly learnt knowledge to check against the statement and structure in existing ontologies. One can apply machine learning (or deep learning) using one version of an ontology as training source and the next version for evaluation; or one can split the same version of an ontology into training and test sets in a cross-validation manner; or one can learn from the entire UMLS to obtain a trained model and apply it for validating statements or "facts" captured in domain specific ontologies (taking it out of the training set, if relevant).

The possibilities seem to be wide-ranging, although all approaches would involve two key ingredients: embedding of a graph or an ordered structure, and embedding of concept labels and declarative statements. For instance, Liu et al. [113] have explored the feasibility of using Doc2Vec to obtain embeddings for concepts and a convolutional neural network model to predict missing *is-a* relations in the NCIt. However, their results were not yet practical: when the trained model was used to detect actual missing *is-a* relations (only 1 out of 20 random suggestions were valid). Another challenge in using such learning-based methods is the selection or generation of training samples, such as how to choose negative samples to train a classification model for the *is-a* prediction task. The typical sample imbalance scenario arises here as well. Further research is needed to explore machine learning-based approaches for biomedical ontologies in comparison with the formal method-based approaches covered in the book.

Appendix

Ontological Resources

SNOMED CT.

SNOMED International, a not-for-profit organization registered in England and Wales, is the company that owns, administers and develops SNOMED CT. The main website is www.snomed.org. There is no charge for SNOMED International Member countries or territories for use of SNOMED CT. The SNOMED CT United States Edition is managed by the U.S. National Library of Medicine and downloadable from www.nlm.nih.gov/healthit/snomedct. As a Member country, use of SNOMED CT in the U.S. is free of charge. SNOMED CT Browser (browser.ihtsdotools.org) provides localized interfaces in the respective languages for exploring the content of SNOMED CT. Though not a graphical rendering engine for inspecting the structure, the browser allows a user to look up definitions and navigate hierarchies using the parent-child up-down modality.

Gene Ontology.

The GO is managed by the Gene Ontology Consortium, a large, international group of scientists in the disciplines of biology and computer science, with the mission "to develop a comprehensive, computational

© The Editor(s) (if applicable) and The Author(s), under exclusive license to Springer
Nature Switzerland AG 2022
G.-Q. Zhang et al., *Formal Methods for the Analysis of Biomedical Ontologies*,
Synthesis Lectures on Data, Semantics, and Knowledge,
https://doi.org/10.1007/978-3-031-12131-9

model of biological systems, ranging from the molecular to the organism level, across the multiplicity of species in the tree of life." The Gene Ontology Consortium's main website, geneontology.org, provides the GO and associated resources and tools for its use.

NCI Thesaurus.   The NCIt can be accessed through NCI's website ncithesaurus.nci.nih.gov. It is produced and managed by NCI Enterprise Vocabulary Services (EVS), a collaborative effort of the NCI Office of Communications and the NCI Center for Bioinformatics. The EVS provides a set of services and resources, including NCI Thesaurus and NCI Metathesaurus, that facilitate the standardization of terminology across the Institute and the larger biomedical community, including the Clinical Data Interchange Standards Consortium Terminology (CDISC), the U.S. Food and Drug Administration (FDA), the Federal Medication Terminologies (FMT), and the National Council for Prescription Drug Programs (NCPDP).

Unified Medical Language System.   The UMLS is managed by the U.S. National Library of Medicine (www.nlm.nih.gov/research/umls). Training and documentation, as well as local installation guide are provided. There is no charge for licensing the UMLS from NLM for use in the United States and other SNOMED International member countries.

BioPortal.   The BioPortal is a comprehensive repository of biomedical ontologies. This is the resource for finding and using special-purpose and domain-specific ontologies developed and shared by the community. Led by Dr. Mark Musen, the Stanford's Center for Biomedical Informatics Research (BMIR) team supports the BioPortal software and performs all modifications, system operations, user support, and outreach activities.

Protégé.   A free, open-source ontology editor, Protégé (protege.stanford.edu) is also developed by the same Stanford team (see previous item).

Web Ontology Language.   OWL is a standard formal language for ontology specification, representation, and distribution, developed by the World Wide Web Consortium (W3C).

Sample Hasse Diagrams of Non-lattice Subgraphs and Suggested Remediations (SNOMED CT September 2015 US edition)

1. Revision of dacryocystorhinostomy and insertion of tube
    is-a
    Revision of dacryocystorhinostomy

Non-lattice Subgraph:

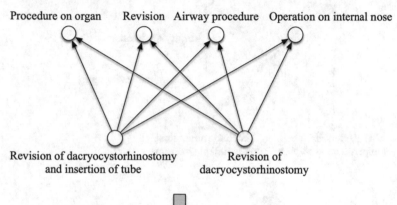

Suggested remediation:

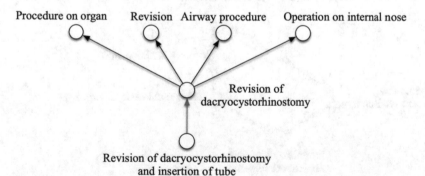

Rationale: The concept *"Revision of dacryocystorhinostomy and insertion of tube"* is a specific case of *"Revision of dacryocystorhinostomy"* where "insertion of tub" is involved. Hence, the former concept should be a subtype of the latter.

2. Traumatic abdominal compartment syndrome
   is-a
   Abdominal compartment syndrome

Non-lattice Subgraph:

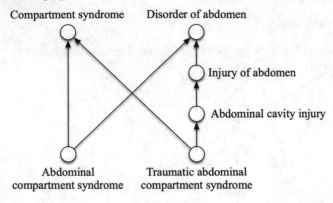

Suggested remediation:

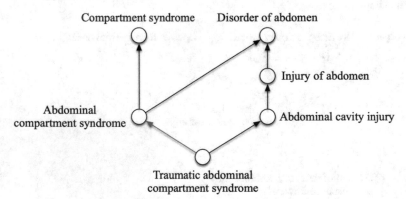

Rationale: The modifier "Traumatic" in the concept "*Traumatic abdominal compartment syndrome*" makes it a specific case of "*Abdominal compartment syndrome.*" Therefore, the former concept should be a subtype of the latter.

3. Lumbar spondylosis with myelopathy
   is-a
   Lumbar spondylosis

Non-lattice Subgraph:

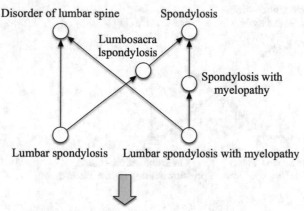

Suggested remediation:

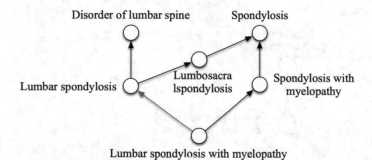

Rationale: The concept "*Lumbar spondylosis with myelopathy*" discusses a specific case of "*Lumbar spondylosis*" that includes "myelopathy." Hence, the former concept should be a subtype of the latter.

4. On examination - blood pressure reading low
   is-a
   Low blood pressure reading

Non-lattice Subgraph:

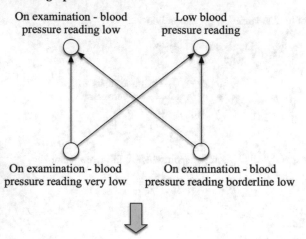

Suggested remediation:

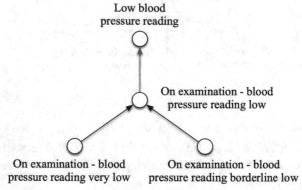

Rationale: The concept "*On examination - blood pressure reading low*" due to the part "On examination" is a specific case of "*Low blood pressure reading*." Therefore, the former concept should be a subtype of the latter.

5. Bilateral intermittent exotropia
   is-a
   Intermittent exotropia

Non-lattice Subgraph:

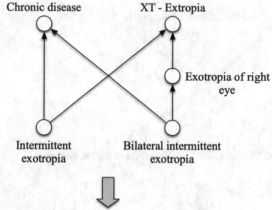

Suggested remediation:

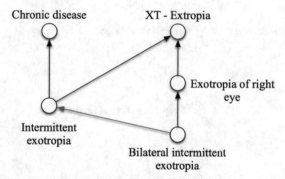

Rationale: The modifier "Bilateral" in the concept "*Bilateral intermittent exotropia*" makes it a specific case of "*Intermittent exotropia.*" Therefore the former concept is a subtype of the latter.

6. Deep laceration of nail of finger
   is-a
   Deep laceration of finger

Non-lattice Subgraph:

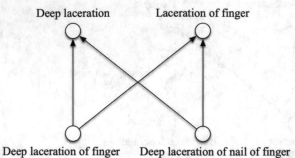

Suggested remediation:

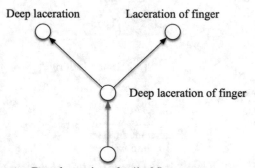

Rationale: The fact that "*Deep laceration of nail of finger*" is both a subtype of "*Deep laceration*" and a subtype of "*Laceration of finger*" implies that "*Deep laceration of nail of finger*" should be a subtype of "*Deep laceration of finger.*"

7. Cecostomy tube procedure using fluoroscopic guidance
   is-a
   Cecostomy using fluoroscopic guidance

Non-lattice Subgraph:

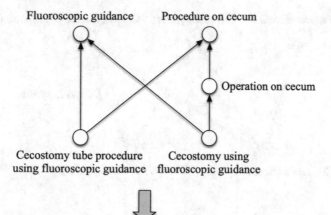

Suggested remediation:

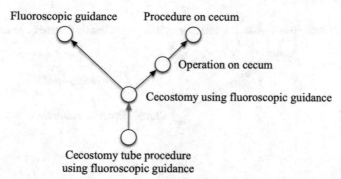

Rationale: The addition of "tube procedure" to the concept "*Cecostomy tube procedure using fluoroscopic guidance*" makes it a more specific case of "*Cecostomy using fluoroscopic guidance.*" Therefore, the former concept should be a subtype of the latter.

8. Recurrent infective cystitis
   is-a
   Chronic infective cystitis

Non-lattice Subgraph:

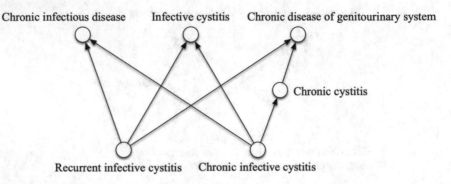

Suggested remediation:

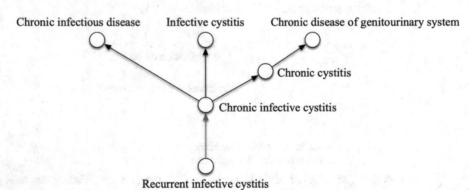

Rationale: The existing relation "*Recurrent infective cystitis*" *is-a* "*Chronic infectious disease*" implies that the former concept is a "chronic disease." Therefore, "*Recurrent infective cystitis*" should be a subtype of "*Chronic infective cystitis.*"

9. Acute endometritis
   is-a
   Acute uterine inflammatory disease

Non-lattice Subgraph:

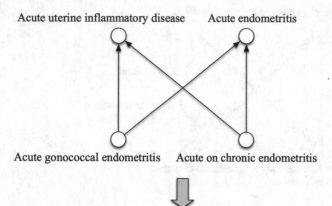

Suggested remediation:

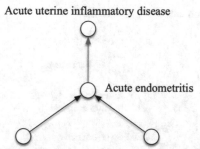

Rationale: The existing relation "*Acute on chronic endometritis*" *is-a* "*Acute uterine inflammatory disease*" implies that "endometritis" is a subtype of "uterine inflammatory disease". Therefore, "*Acute endometritis*" should be a subtype of "*Acute uterine inflammatory disease.*"

10. Removal of foreign body of cornea by incision
    is-a
    Incision of cornea

Non-lattice Subgraph:

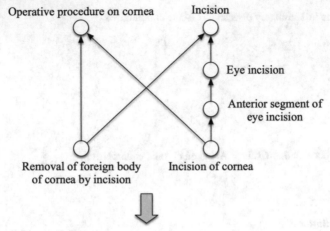

Suggested remediation:

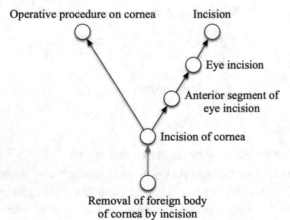

Rationale: The concept "*Removal of foreign body of cornea by incision*" is a specific case of "*Incision of cornea*" performed to remove a "foreign body" from the "cornea."

11. Basal cell carcinoma of skin of lip
    is-a
    Carcinoma of lip

Non-lattice Subgraph:

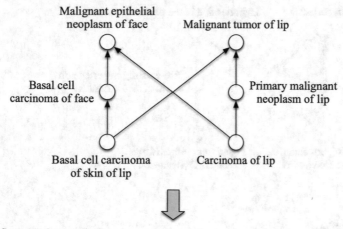

Suggested remediation:

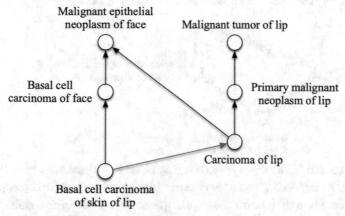

Rationale: "Basal cell carcinoma" is a subtype of "carcinoma" and "skin of lip" is a part of "lip." These imply that concept *Basal cell carcinoma of skin of lip* should be a subtype of *Carcinoma of lip*.

12. Postpartum pre-existing essential hypertension
    is-a
    Essential hypertension in obstetric context

Non-lattice Subgraph:

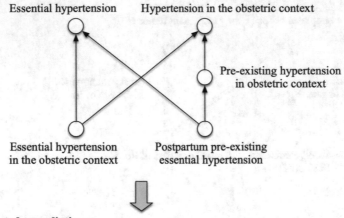

Suggested remediation:

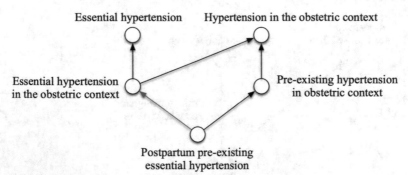

Rationale: The fact that "*Postpartum pre-existing essential hypertension*" is both a subtype of "*Essential hypertension*" and a subtype of "*Hypertension in obstetric context*" implies that it should be a subtype of "*Essential hypertension in obstetric context.*"

13. Intracranial granuloma
    is-a
    Inflammatory disease of the central nervous system

Non-lattice Subgraph:

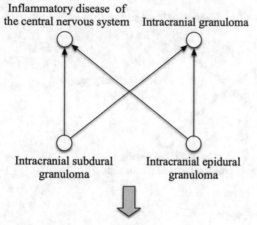

Suggested remediation:

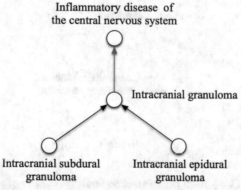

Rationale: The existing relations "*Intracranial epidural granuloma*" *is-a* "*Inflammatory disease of the central nervous system*" and "*Intracranial subdural granuloma*" *is-a* "*Inflammatory disease of the central nervous system*" imply that "*Intracranial granuloma*" should be a subtype of "*Inflammatory disease of the central nervous system.*"

14. Congenital pigmented melanocytic nevus of skin
    is-a
    Congenital hamartoma of skin

Non-lattice Subgraph:

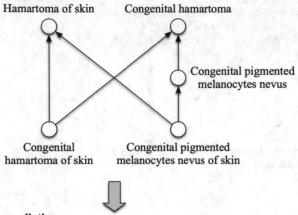

Suggested remediation:

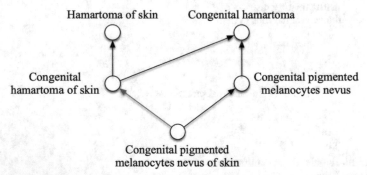

Rationale: The fact that "*Congenital pigmented melanocytic nevus of skin*" is both a subtype of "*Congenital hamartoma*" and a subtype of "*Hamartoma of skin*" implies that "*Congenital pigmented melanocytic nevus of skin*" should be a subtype of "*Congenital hamartoma of skin*."

15. Subcutaneous drug therapy
    is-a
    Drug therapy

Non-lattice Subgraph:

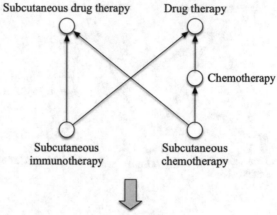

Suggested remediation:

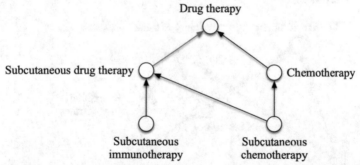

Rationale: The modifier "Subcutaneous" in the concept"*Subcutaneous drug therapy*" implies that "*Subcutaneous drug therapy*" is a specific kind of "*Drug therapy.*" Therefore, "*Subcutaneous drug therapy*" should be a subtype of "*Drug therapy.*"

16. Superficial injury of chest
    is-a
    Chest injury

Non-lattice Subgraph:

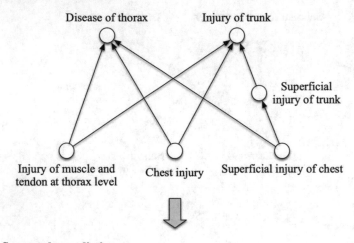

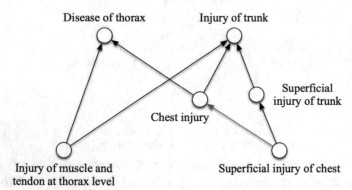

Rationale: "Superficial injury" is a kind of "injury." Hence, the concept "*Superficial injury of chest*" should be a subtype of "*Chest injury*."

17. Acromioclavicular joint pain
    is-a
    Shoulder joint pain

Non-lattice Subgraph:

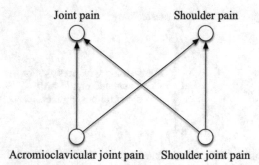

Joint pain   Shoulder pain

Acromioclavicular joint pain   Shoulder joint pain

Suggested remediation:

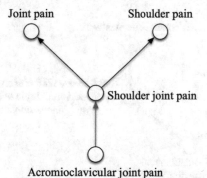

Joint pain   Shoulder pain

Shoulder joint pain

Acromioclavicular joint pain

Rationale: The fact that "*Acromioclavicular joint pain*" is both a subtype of "*Shoulder pain*" and "*Joint pain*" implies that it should be a subtype of "*Shoulder joint pain*."

18. Bilateral subcutaneous mammectomy with synchronous implant
    is-a
    Bilateral subcutaneous mammectomy

Non-lattice Subgraph:

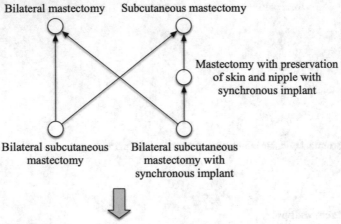

Suggested remediation:

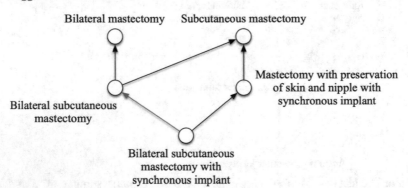

Rationale: "*Bilateral subcutaneous mammectomy with synchronous implant*" is a specific type of "*Bilateral subcutaneous mammectomy*" where a "synchronous implant" is involved. Therefore, the former concept should be a subtype of the latter.

19. Neonatal cardiorespiratory arrest
    is-a
    Cardiorespiratory arrest

Non-lattice Subgraph:

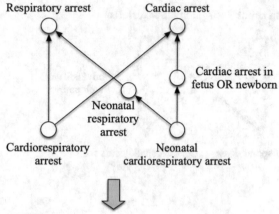

Suggested remediation:

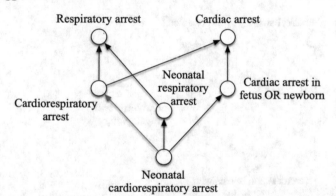

Rationale: The modifier "Neonatal" implies that the concept "*Neonatal cardiorespiratory arrest*" is a specific type of "*Cardiorespiratory arrest.*" Therefore, the former concept should be a subtype of the latter.

20. Cervical spondylosis with myelopathy
    is-a
    Cervical spondylosis

Non-lattice Subgraph:

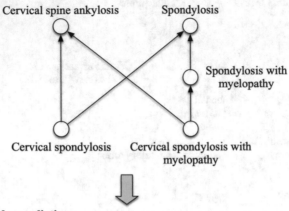

Suggested remediation:

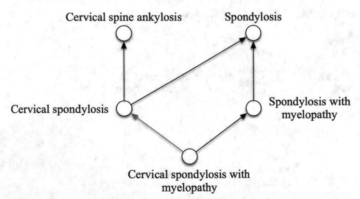

Rationale: "*Cervical spondylosis with myelopathy*" is a specific type of "*Cervical spondylosis*" where "myelopathy" is involved. Therefore, the former concept should be a subtype of the latter.

References

1. Benjamin Carlson. Quote of the Day: Google CEO Compares Data Across Millennia. https://www.theatlantic.com/technology/archive/2010/07/quote-of-the-day-google-ceo-compares-data-across-millennia/344989/, 2010. [Online; Accessed 28 Apr 2022].
2. Olivier Bodenreider. The unified medical language system (umls): integrating biomedical terminology. *Nucleic acids research*, 32(suppl_1):D267–D270, 2004.
3. Natalya F Noy, Nigam H Shah, Patricia L Whetzel, Benjamin Dai, Michael Dorf, Nicholas Griffith, Clement Jonquet, Daniel L Rubin, Margaret-Anne Storey, Christopher G Chute, et al. Bioportal: ontologies and integrated data resources at the click of a mouse. *Nucleic acids research*, 37(suppl_2):W170–W173, 2009.
4. The National Center for Biomedical Ontology. Welcome to BioPortal, the world's most comprehensive repository of biomedical ontologies. https://bioportal.bioontology.org/, 2021. [Accessed Aprill-2022].
5. Mark D Wilkinson, Michel Dumontier, IJsbrand Jan Aalbersberg, Gabrielle Appleton, Myles Axton, Arie Baak, Niklas Blomberg, Jan-Willem Boiten, Luiz Bonino da Silva Santos, Philip E Bourne, et al. The fair guiding principles for scientific data management and stewardship. *Scientific data*, 3(1):1–9, 2016.
6. Russell L Ackoff. From data to wisdom. *Journal of applied systems analysis*, 16(1):3–9, 1989.
7. Kevin Donnelly. SNOMED-CT: The advanced terminology and coding system for eHealth. *Studies in health technology and informatics*, 121:279, 2006.
8. Michael Ashburner, Catherine A Ball, Judith A Blake, David Botstein, Heather Butler, J Michael Cherry, Allan P Davis, Kara Dolinski, Selina S Dwight, Janan T Eppig, et al. Gene ontology: tool for the unification of biology. *Nature genetics*, 25(1):25, 2000.
9. Nicholas Sioutos, Sherri de Coronado, Margaret W Haber, Frank W Hartel, Wen-Ling Shaiu, and Lawrence W Wright. Nci thesaurus: a semantic model integrating cancer-related clinical and molecular information. *Journal of biomedical informatics*, 40(1):30–43, 2007.
10. Cornelius Rosse and Jose LV Mejino. The foundational model of anatomy ontology. In *Anatomy Ontologies for Bioinformatics*, pages 59–117. Springer, 2008.
11. SNOMED International. Snomed international. https://www.snomed.org/, 2020. [Online; Accessed 2 May 2022].

© The Editor(s) (if applicable) and The Author(s), under exclusive license to Springer Nature Switzerland AG 2022
G.-Q. Zhang et al., *Formal Methods for the Analysis of Biomedical Ontologies*, Synthesis Lectures on Data, Semantics, and Knowledge, https://doi.org/10.1007/978-3-031-12131-9

12. SNOMED International. Snomed ct global clinical terminology is introduced in germany through the meidical informatics initiative. https://www.snomed.org/news-and-events/articles/snomedct-introduced-in-germany-through-MII#::text=Owned%20and%20maintained%20by%20SNOMED,in%20research%20and%20planning%20capacities. 2020. [Online; Accessed 2 May 2022].

13. SNOMED International. directed acyclic graph. https://confluence.ihtsdotools.org/display/DOCGLOSS/directed+acyclic+graph, 2022. [Online; Accessed 2 May 2022].

14. SNOMED International. Domain specific modeling. https://confluence.ihtsdotools.org/display/DOCEG/Domain+Specific+Modeling#::text=SNOMED%20CT%20is%20arranged%20as,above%20them%20in%20a%20hierarchy. 2022. [Online; Accessed 2 May 2022].

15. SNOMED International. Description logic over terminology. https://confluence.ihtsdotools.org/display/DOCANLYT/6.4+Description+Logic+Over+Terminology#::text=SNOMED%20CT's%20semantics%20are%20based,possible%20using%20most%20other%20approaches. 2022. [Online; Accessed 2 May 2022].

16. SNOMED International. SNOMED International SNOMED CT Browser. https://browser.ihtsdotools.org/, 2022. [Online; Accessed 2 May 2022].

17. Gene Ontology Consortium. Gene Ontology Overview. http://geneontology.org/docs/ontology-documentation/, 2022. [Online; Accessed 2 May 2022].

18. Haiming Tang, Christopher J Mungall, Huaiyu Mi, and Paul D Thomas. Gotaxon: representing the evolution of biological functions in the gene ontology. *arXiv preprint* arXiv:1802.06004, 2018.

19. Sherri de Coronado, Lawrence W Wright, Gilberto Fragoso, Margaret W Haber, Elizabeth A Hahn-Dantona, Francis W Hartel, Sharon L Quan, Tracy Safran, Nicole Thomas, and Lori Whiteman. The nci thesaurus quality assurance life cycle. *Journal of biomedical informatics*, 42(3):530–539, 2009.

20. Enterprise Vocabulary Services. NCI Thesaurus Hierarchy. https://ncit.nci.nih.gov/ncitbrowser/pages/hierarchy.jsf?dictionary=NCI_Thesaurus&version=22.04d, 2022. [Online; Accessed 2 May 2022].

21. Dieter Fensel. Ontologies. In *Ontologies*, pages 11–18. Springer, 2001.

22. Gianluigi Greco, Marco Manna, and Francesco Ricca. Ontology: Introduction. In Shoba Ranganathan, Michael Gribskov, Kenta Nakai, and Christian Schönbach, editors, *Encyclopedia of Bioinformatics and Computational Biology*, pages 785–789. Academic Press, Oxford, January 2019.

23. Wolfram MathWorld. Hasse Diagram. https://mathworld.wolfram.com/HasseDiagram.html, 2022. [Online; Accessed 3 May 2022].

24. Alan Jovic, Marin Prcela, and Dragan Gamberger. Ontologies in medical knowledge representation. In *2007 29th International Conference on Information Technology Interfaces*, pages 535–540. IEEE, 2007.

25. James J Cimino. Desiderata for controlled medical vocabularies in the twenty-first century. *Methods of information in medicine*, 37(04/05):394–403, 1998.

26. Songmao Zhang and Olivier Bodenreider. Law and order: Assessing and enforcing compliance with ontological modeling principles in the foundational model of anatomy. *Computers in Biology and Medicine*, 36(7-8):674–693, 2006.

27. Dmitry I Ignatov. Introduction to formal concept analysis and its applications in information retrieval and related fields. In *Russian Summer School in Information Retrieval*, pages 42–141. Springer, 2014.

28. Xinxin Zhu, Jung-Wei Fan, David M Baorto, Chunhua Weng, and James J Cimino. A review of auditing methods applied to the content of controlled biomedical terminologies. *Journal of biomedical informatics*, 42(3):413–425, 2009.

29. Ling Zheng, Zhe He, Duo Wei, Vipina Keloth, Jung-Wei Fan, Luke Lindemann, Xinxin Zhu, James J Cimino, and Yehoshua Perl. A review of auditing techniques for the unified medical language system. *Journal of the American Medical Informatics Association*, 27(10):1625–1638, 2020.

30. Muhammad F Amith, Zhe He, Jiang Bian, Juan Antonio Lossio-Ventura, and Cui Tao. Assessing the practice of biomedical ontology evaluation: Gaps and opportunities. *Journal of biomedical informatics*, 2018.

31. Natalya Fridman Noy, Monica Crubézy, Ray W Fergerson, Holger Knublauch, Samson W Tu, Jennifer Vendetti, and Mark A Musen. Protégé-2000: an open-source ontology-development and knowledge-acquisition environment. In *AMIA Annual Symposium Proceedings*, volume 2003, pages 953–953. American Medical Informatics Association, 2003.

32. Michael Sintek. OntoViz. https://protegewiki.stanford.edu/wiki/OntoViz, 2022. [Online; Accessed 3 May 2022].

33. Harith Alani. Tgviztab: an ontology visualisation extension for protégé. In *Workshop on Visualization Information in Knowledge Engineering*, 2003.

34. Margaret-Anne Storey, Casey Best, Jeff Michaud, Derek Rayside, Marin Litoiu, and Mark Musen. Shrimp views: an interactive environment for information visualization and navigation. In *CHI'02 Extended Abstracts on Human Factors in Computing Systems*, pages 520–521. ACM, 2002.

35. Margaret-Anne Storey, Mark Musen, John Silva, Casey Best, Neil Ernst, Ray Fergerson, and Natasha Noy. Jambalaya: Interactive visualization to enhance ontology authoring and knowledge acquisition in protégé. In *Workshop on interactive tools for knowledge capture*, volume 73, page 12. Citeseer, 2001.

36. Peter Eklund, Nataliya Roberts, and Steve Green. Ontorama: Browsing rdf ontologies using a hyperbolic-style browser. In *First International Symposium on Cyber Worlds, 2002. Proceedings.*, pages 405–411. IEEE, 2002.

37. Alessio Bosca, Dario Bonino, and Paolo Pellegrino. Ontosphere: more than a 3d ontology visualization tool. In *Swap*. Citeseer, 2005.

38. Christopher Ochs, James Geller, Yehoshua Perl, and Mark A Musen. A unified software framework for deriving, visualizing, and exploring abstraction networks for ontologies. *Journal of biomedical informatics*, 62:90–105, 2016.

39. Michael Hartung, Toralf Kirsten, Anika Gross, and Erhard Rahm. Onex: Exploring changes in life science ontologies. *BMC bioinformatics*, 10(1):1–10, 2009.

40. Werner Ceusters. Applying evolutionary terminology auditing to snomed ct. In *AMIA annual symposium proceedings*, volume 2010, page 96. American Medical Informatics Association, 2010.

41. Shiqiang Tao, Licong Cui, Wei Zhu, Mengmeng Sun, Olivier Bodenreider, and Guo-Qiang Zhang. Mining relation reversals in the evolution of snomed ct using mapreduce. *AMIA Summits on Translational Science Proceedings*, 2015:46, 2015.

42. EA Mendona, James J Cimino, Keith E Campbell, and Kent A Spackman. Reproducibility of interpreting and" and" or" in terminology systems. In *Proceedings of the AMIA Symposium*, page 790. American Medical Informatics Association, 1998.

43. Robert H Dolin, Stanley M Huff, Roberto A Rocha, Kent A Spackman, and Keith E Campbell. Evaluation of a "lexically assign, logically refine" strategy for semi-automated integration of overlapping terminologies. *Journal of the American Medical Informatics Association*, 5(2):203–213, 1998.

44. Francisco M Couto, Mário J Silva, and Pedro M Coutinho. Measuring semantic similarity between gene ontology terms. *Data & knowledge engineering*, 61(1):137–152, 2007.
45. Fausto Giunchiglia, Aliaksandr Autayeu, and Juan Pane. S-match: an open source framework for matching lightweight ontologies. *Semantic Web*, 3(3):307–317, 2012.
46. R Sedgewick and K Wayne. Algorithms, 2011, 2001.
47. Thomas H Cormen, Charles E Leiserson, Ronald L Rivest, and Clifford Stein. Section 22.4: Topological sort. *Introduction to Algorithms (2nd ed.), MIT Press and McGraw-Hill*, pages 549–552, 2001.
48. Guangming Xing, Guo-Qiang Zhang, and Licong Cui. Fedrr: fast, exhaustive detection of redundant hierarchical relations for quality improvement of large biomedical ontologies. *BioData mining*, 9(1):31, 2016.
49. Olivier Bodenreider. Strength in numbers: exploring redundancy in hierarchical relations across biomedical terminologies. In *AMIA*, 2003.
50. Huanying Helen Gu, Duo Wei, Jose LV Mejino, and Gai Elhanan. Relationship auditing of the fma ontology. *Journal of biomedical informatics*, 42(3):550–557, 2009.
51. Fleur Mougin. Identifying redundant and missing relations in the gene ontology. In *MIE*, pages 195–199, 2015.
52. Fleur Mougin and Natalia Grabar. Auditing the multiply-related concepts within the umls. *Journal of the American Medical Informatics Association*, 21(e2):e185–e193, 2014.
53. Huanying Gu, Gai Elhanan, Michael Halper, and Zhe He. Questionable relationship triples in the umls. In *Biomedical and Health Informatics (BHI), 2012 IEEE-EMBS International Conference on*, pages 713–716. IEEE, 2012.
54. O. Bodenreider. Circular hierarchical relationships in the umls: etiology, diagnosis, treatment, complications and prevention. In *Proceedings of the AMIA Symposium*, pages 57–61, 2001.
55. F Mougin and O Bodenreider. Approaches to eliminating cycles in the umls metathesaurus: naive vs. formal. In *Proceedings of the AMIA Symposium*, pages 550–554, 2005.
56. M Halper, CP Morrey, Y Chen, G Elhanan, G Hripcsak, and Y Perl. Auditing hierarchical cycles to locate other inconsistencies in the umls. In *Proceedings of the AMIA Symposium*, pages 529–536, 2011.
57. Licong Cui. Cohere: Cross-ontology hierarchical relation examination for ontology quality assurance. *AMIA Annual Symp Proc*, 2015:2092–2100, 2015.
58. Cornelius Rosse and José LV Mejino Jr. A reference ontology for biomedical informatics: the foundational model of anatomy. *Journal of biomedical informatics*, 36(6):478–500, 2003.
59. Rainer Beck and Stefan Schulz. Logic-based remodeling of the digital anatomist foundational model. In *AMIA Annual Symposium Proceedings*, volume 2003, page 71. American Medical Informatics Association, 2003.
60. World Wide Web Consortium. SPARQL. http://www.w3.org/TR/rdf-sparql-query/, 2012. [Accessed 20-October-2012].
61. OpenLink Software. Virtuoso. http://virtuoso.openlinksw.com/, 2012. [Accessed 20-October-2012].
62. Guo-Qiang Zhang, Lingyun Luo, Chime Ogbuji, Cliff Joslyn, Jose Mejino, and Satya S Sahoo. An analysis of multi-type relational interactions in fma using graph motifs with disjointness constraints. In *AMIA Annual Symposium Proceedings*, volume 2012, page 1060. American Medical Informatics Association, 2012.
63. Gongqing Zhang. *Logic of domains*. Springer Science & Business Media, 2012.
64. Olivier Dameron, Daniel L Rubin, and Mark A Musen. Challenges in converting frame-based ontology into owl: the foundational model of anatomy case-study. In *AMIA Annual Symposium Proceedings*, volume 2005, page 181. American Medical Informatics Association, 2005.

65. Cliff Joslyn, Sinan al Saffar, David Haglin, and Lawrence Holder. Combinatorial information theoretical measurement of the semantic significance of semantic graph motifs. In *Proceedings of the Mining Data Semantic Workshop (MDS 2011), SIGKDD*. Citeseer, 2011.

66. Robin Milner. A complete inference system for a class of regular behaviours. *Journal of Computer and System Sciences*, 28(3):439–466, 1984.

67. Lingyun Luo. An effective coalgebraic bisimulation proof method. *Electronic Notes in Theoretical Computer Science*, 164(1):105–119, 2006.

68. Olivier Dameron, Mark A Musen, and Bernard Gibaud. Using semantic dependencies for consistency management of an ontology of brain–cortex anatomy. *Artificial Intelligence in Medicine*, 39(3):217–225, 2007.

69. Jonathan M Mortensen, Matthew Horridge, Mark A Musen, and Natalya F Noy. Applications of ontology design patterns in biomedical ontologies. In *AMIA Annual Symposium Proceedings*, volume 2012, page 643. American Medical Informatics Association, 2012.

70. Lingyun Luo, José LV Mejino Jr, and Guo-Qiang Zhang. An analysis of fma using structural self-bisimilarity. *Journal of biomedical informatics*, 46(3):497–505, 2013.

71. Hua Min, Yehoshua Perl, Yan Chen, Michael Halper, James Geller, and Yue Wang. Auditing as part of the terminology design life cycle. *Journal of the American Medical Informatics Association*, 13(6):676–690, 2006.

72. The OBO Foundry. The Open Biological and Biomedical Ontology (OBO) Foundry. http://www.obofoundry.org/cgi-bin/detail.cgi?id=fma_lite, 2012. [Accessed 20-October-2012].

73. National Library of Medicine. Lexical tools: Luinorm. https://lexsrv3.nlm.nih.gov/LexSysGroup/Projects/lvg/2020/docs/userDoc/tools/luiNorm.html, 2020. [Accessed Oct-2020].

74. Adam D Troy, Guo-Qiang Zhang, and Ye Tian. Faster concept analysis. In *International Conference on Conceptual Structures*, pages 206–219. Springer, 2007.

75. Fengbo Zheng and Licong Cui. A lexical-based formal concept analysis method to identify missing concepts in the nci thesaurus. In *2020 IEEE International Conference on Bioinformatics and Biomedicine (BIBM)*, pages 1757–1760. IEEE, 2020.

76. Guoqian Jiang and Christopher G Chute. Auditing the semantic completeness of snomed ct using formal concept analysis. *Journal of the American Medical Informatics Association*, 16(1):89–102, 2009.

77. Sergei O Kuznetsov and Sergei A Obiedkov. Comparing performance of algorithms for generating concept lattices. *Journal of Experimental & Theoretical Artificial Intelligence*, 14(2-3):189–216, 2002.

78. Jean-Paul Bordat. Calcul pratique du treillis de galois d'une correspondance. *Mathématiques et Sciences humaines*, 96:31–47, 1986.

79. Michel Chein. Algorithme de recherche des sous-matrices premières d'une matrice. *Bulletin mathématique de la Société des Sciences Mathématiques de la République Socialiste de Roumanie*, pages 21–25, 1969.

80. Wei Zhu, Licong Cui, and Guo-Qiang Zhang. Spark-mca: Large-scale, exhaustive formal concept analysis for evaluating the semantic completeness of snomed ct. In *AMIA Annual Symposium Proceedings*, volume 2017, page 1931. American Medical Informatics Association, 2017.

81. Pierre Zweigenbaum, Bruno Bachimont, Jacques Bouaud, Jean Charlet, Jean-François Boisvieux, et al. Issues in the structuring and acquisition of an ontology for medical language understanding. *Methods of information in medicine*, 34:15–15, 1995.

82. Bernhard Ganter and Rudolf Wille. *Formal concept analysis: mathematical foundations*. Springer Science & Business Media, 2012.

83. Guo-Qiang Zhang and Olivier Bodenreider. Large-scale, exhaustive lattice-based structural auditing of snomed ct. In *AMIA Annual Symposium Proceedings*, volume 2010, page 922. American Medical Informatics Association, 2010.

84. Guo-Qiang Zhang and Olivier Bodenreider. Using sparql to test for lattices: application to quality assurance in biomedical ontologies. In *International Semantic Web Conference*, pages 273–288. Springer, 2010.

85. Jeffrey Dean and Sanjay Ghemawat. Mapreduce: simplified data processing on large clusters. *Communications of the ACM*, 51(1):107–113, 2008.

86. Licong Cui, Shiqiang Tao, and Guo-Qiang Zhang. Biomedical ontology quality assurance using a big data approach. *ACM Transactions on Knowledge Discovery from Data (TKDD)*, 10(4):41, 2016.

87. Guo-Qiang Zhang, Wei Zhu, Mengmeng Sun, Shiqiang Tao, Olivier Bodenreider, and Licong Cui. Maple: a mapreduce pipeline for lattice-based evaluation and its application to snomed ct. In *2014 IEEE International Conference on Big Data (Big Data)*, pages 754–759. IEEE, 2014.

88. Yue Wang, Michael Halper, Hua Min, Yehoshua Perl, Yan Chen, and Kent A Spackman. Structural methodologies for auditing snomed. *Journal of biomedical informatics*, 40(5):561–581, 2007.

89. Alan L Rector, Jeremy E Rogers, and Pam Pole. The galen high level ontology. In *Medical Informatics Europe'96*, pages 174–178. IOS Press, 1996.

90. Camil Demetrescu and Giuseppe F Italiano. Fully dynamic transitive closure: breaking through the o (n/sup 2/) barrier. In *Proceedings 41st Annual Symposium on Foundations of Computer Science*, pages 381–389. IEEE, 2000.

91. Zvi Galil and Giuseppe F Italiano. Data structures and algorithms for disjoint set union problems. *ACM Computing Surveys (CSUR)*, 23(3):319–344, 1991.

92. Guo-Qiang Zhang, Guangming Xing, and Licong Cui. An efficient, large-scale, non-lattice-detection algorithm for exhaustive structural auditing of biomedical ontologies. *Journal of biomedical informatics*, 80:106–119, 2018.

93. Michael A Bender, Martin Farach-Colton, Giridhar Pemmasani, Steven Skiena, and Pavel Sumazin. Lowest common ancestors in trees and directed acyclic graphs. *Journal of Algorithms*, 57(2):75–94, 2005.

94. Artur Czumaj, Mirosław Kowaluk, and Andrzej Lingas. Faster algorithms for finding lowest common ancestors in directed acyclic graphs. *Theoretical Computer Science*, 380(1-2):37–46, 2007.

95. Santanu Kumar Dash, Sven-Bodo Scholz, Stephan Herhut, and Bruce Christianson. A scalable approach to computing representative lowest common ancestor in directed acyclic graphs. *Theoretical Computer Science*, 513:25–37, 2013.

96. Stefan Eckhardt, Andreas Michael Mühling, and Johannes Nowak. Fast lowest common ancestor computations in dags. In *European Symposium on Algorithms*, pages 705–716. Springer, 2007.

97. Wei Zhu, Guo-Qiang Zhang, Shiqiang Tao, Mengmeng Sun, and Licong Cui. Neo: systematic non-lattice embedding of ontologies for comparing the subsumption relationship in snomed ct and in fma using mapreduce. *AMIA Summits on Translational Science Proceedings*, 2015:216, 2015.

98. Licong Cui, Wei Zhu, Shiqiang Tao, James T Case, Olivier Bodenreider, and Guo-Qiang Zhang. Mining non-lattice subgraphs for detecting missing hierarchical relations and concepts in SNOMED CT. *Journal of the American Medical Informatics Association*, 24(4):788–798, 2017.

99. Rashmie Abeysinghe, Michael A Brooks, Jeffery Talbert, and Licong Cui. Quality assurance of nci thesaurus by mining structural-lexical patterns. In *AMIA Annual Symposium Proceedings*, volume 2017, page 364. American Medical Informatics Association, 2017.

100. Olivier Bodenreider, Anita Burgun, and Thomas C Rindflesch. Assessing the consistency of a biomedical terminology through lexical knowledge. *International journal of medical informatics*, 67(1-3):85–95, 2002.

101. Ankur Agrawal and Gai Elhanan. Contrasting lexical similarity and formal definitions in snomed ct: consistency and implications. *Journal of biomedical informatics*, 47:192–198, 2014.

102. Alan Rector and Luigi Iannone. Lexically suggest, logically define: Quality assurance of the use of qualifiers and expected results of post-coordination in snomed ct. *Journal of biomedical informatics*, 45(2):199–209, 2012.

103. Yue Wang, Michael Halper, Duo Wei, Yehoshua Perl, and James Geller. Abstraction of complex concepts with a refined partial-area taxonomy of snomed. *Journal of biomedical informatics*, 45(1):15–29, 2012.

104. Yue Wang, Michael Halper, Duo Wei, Huanying Gu, Yehoshua Perl, Junchuan Xu, Gai Elhanan, Yan Chen, Kent A Spackman, James T Case, et al. Auditing complex concepts of snomed using a refined hierarchical abstraction network. *Journal of biomedical informatics*, 45(1):1–14, 2012.

105. Christopher Ochs, James Geller, Yehoshua Perl, Yan Chen, Junchuan Xu, Hua Min, James T Case, and Zhi Wei. Scalable quality assurance for large snomed ct hierarchies using subject-based subtaxonomies. *Journal of the American Medical Informatics Association*, 22(3):507–518, 2015.

106. Christopher Ochs, James Geller, Yehoshua Perl, Yan Chen, Ankur Agrawal, James T Case, and George Hripcsak. A tribal abstraction network for snomed ct target hierarchies without attribute relationships. *Journal of the American Medical Informatics Association*, 22(3):628–639, 2014.

107. George A Miller. Wordnet: a lexical database for english. *Communications of the ACM*, 38(11):39–41, 1995.

108. Princeton University. About WordNet. https://wordnet.princeton.edu/, 2010. [Accessed 15-March-2018].

109. Licong Cui, Olivier Bodenreider, Jay Shi, and Guo-Qiang Zhang. Auditing snomed ct hierarchical relations based on lexical features of concepts in non-lattice subgraphs. *Journal of biomedical informatics*, 78:177–184, 2018.

110. Rashmie Abeysinghe, Michael A Brooks, and Licong Cui. Leveraging non-lattice subgraphs to audit hierarchical relations in nci thesaurus. In *AMIA Annual Symposium Proceedings*, volume 2019. American Medical Informatics Association, 2019.

111. Licong Cui, Rashmie Abeysinghe, Fengbo Zheng, Shiqiang Tao, Ningzhou Zeng, Isaac Hands, Eric B Durbin, Lori Whiteman, Lyubov Remennik, Nicholas Sioutos, et al. Enhancing the quality of hierarchic relations in the national cancer institute thesaurus to enable faceted query of cancer registry data. *JCO clinical cancer informatics*, 4:392–398, 2020.

112. Olivier Bodenreider. Identifying missing hierarchical relations in snomed ct from logical definitions based on the lexical features of concept names. *ICBO/BioCreative*, 2016, 2016.

113. Hao Liu, Ling Zheng, Yehoshua Perl, James Geller, and Gai Elhanan. Can a convolutional neural network support auditing of nci thesaurus neoplasm concepts? In *ICBO*, 2018.

114. Explosion AI. Spacy: Industrial-strength natural language processing. https://spacy.io/, 2020. [Accessed 15-Feb-2020].

115. National Cancer Institute. Nci thesaurus downloads. https://evs.nci.nih.gov/evs-download/thesaurus-downloads, 2020. [Accessed 19-July-2020].

116. Fengbo Zheng, Rashmie Abeysinghe, Nicholas Sioutos, Lori Whiteman, Lyubov Remennik, and Licong Cui. Detecting missing is-a relations in the nci thesaurus using an enhanced hybrid approach. *BMC Medical Informatics and Decision Making*, 20(10):1–11, 2020.

117. Fengbo Zheng, Rashmie Abeysinghe, and Licong Cui. A hybrid method to detect missing hierarchical relations in nci thesaurus. In *2019 IEEE International Conference on Bioinformatics and Biomedicine (BIBM)*, pages 1948–1953. IEEE, 2019.

118. Dimitris Mossialos, Jean-Marie Meyer, Herbert Budzikiewicz, Ulrich Wolff, Nico Koedam, Christine Baysse, Vanamala Anjaiah, and Pierre Cornelis. Quinolobactin, a new siderophore of pseudomonas fluorescens atcc 17400, the production of which is repressed by the cognate pyoverdine. *Applied and environmental Microbiology*, 66(2):487–492, 2000.

119. Rashmie Abeysinghe, Fengbo Zheng, Eugene W Hinderer, Hunter NB Moseley, and Licong Cui. A lexical approach to identifying subtype inconsistencies in biomedical terminologies. In *2018 IEEE International Conference on Bioinformatics and Biomedicine (BIBM)*, pages 1982–1989. IEEE, 2018.

120. Rashmie Abeysinghe, Eugene W Hinderer, Hunter NB Moseley, and Licong Cui. Auditing subtype inconsistencies among gene ontology concepts. In *2017 IEEE International Conference on Bioinformatics and Biomedicine (BIBM)*, pages 1242–1245. IEEE, 2017.

121. Philip V Ogren, K Bretonnel Cohen, George K Acquaah-Mensah, Jens Eberlein, and Lawrence Hunter. The compositional structure of gene ontology terms. In *Biocomputing 2004*, pages 214–225. World Scientific, 2003.

122. Kristina Toutanova, Dan Klein, Christopher D Manning, and Yoram Singer. Feature-rich part-of-speech tagging with a cyclic dependency network. In *Proceedings of the 2003 Conference of the North American Chapter of the Association for Computational Linguistics on Human Language Technology-Volume 1*, pages 173–180. Association for Computational Linguistics, 2003.

123. Rashmie Abeysinghe, Eugene W Hinderer III, Hunter NB Moseley, and Licong Cui. Ssif: Subsumption-based sub-term inference framework to audit gene ontology. *Bioinformatics*, 36(10):3207–3214, 2020.

124. Aric Hagberg, Pieter Swart, and Daniel S Chult. Exploring network structure, dynamics, and function using networkx. Technical report, Los Alamos National Lab.(LANL), Los Alamos, NM (United States), 2008.

125. Fengbo Zheng, Jay Shi, Yuntao Yang, W Jim Zheng, and Licong Cui. A transformation-based method for auditing the is-a hierarchy of biomedical terminologies in the unified medical language system. *Journal of the American Medical Informatics Association*, 27(10):1568–1575, 2020.

126. Christopher D Manning, Mihai Surdeanu, John Bauer, Jenny Rose Finkel, Steven Bethard, and David McClosky. The stanford corenlp natural language processing toolkit. In *Proceedings of 52nd annual meeting of the association for computational linguistics: system demonstrations*, pages 55–60, 2014.

127. Fengbo Zheng, Jay Shi, and Licong Cui. A lexical-based approach for exhaustive detection of missing hierarchical is-a relations in snomed ct. In *AMIA Annual Symposium Proceedings*, volume 2020, page 1392. American Medical Informatics Association, 2020.

128. The Gene Ontology Consortium. Relations in the gene ontology. http://geneontology.org/docs/ontology-relations/, 2022. [Online; Accessed 25 Jan 2022].

129. The OBO Foundry. Relations ontology. http://www.obofoundry.org/ontology/ro.html, 2022. [Online; Accessed 25 Jan 2022].

130. DV Klopfenstein, Liangsheng Zhang, Brent S Pedersen, Fidel Ramírez, Alex Warwick Vesztrocy, Aurélien Naldi, Christopher J Mungall, Jeffrey M Yunes, Olga Botvinnik, Mark Weigel, et al. Goatools: A python library for gene ontology analyses. *Scientific reports*, 8(1):1–17, 2018.

131. Hershel Raff. Cort, cort, b, corticosterone, and now cortistatin: enough already! *Endocrinology*, 157(9):3307–3308, 2016.

132. David Binns, Emily Dimmer, Rachael Huntley, Daniel Barrell, Claire O'donovan, and Rolf Apweiler. Quickgo: a web-based tool for gene ontology searching. *Bioinformatics*, 25(22):3045–3046, 2009.

133. Rashmie Abeysinghe, Yuntao Yang, Mason Bartels, W Jim Zheng, and Licong Cui. An evidence-based lexical pattern approach for quality assurance of Gene Ontology relations. *Briefings in Bioinformatics*, 04 2022. bbac122.

134. Ankur Agrawal, Yehoshua Perl, Chris Ochs, and Gai Elhanan. Algorithmic detection of inconsistent modeling among snomed ct concepts by combining lexical and structural indicators. In *Bioinformatics and Biomedicine (BIBM), 2015 IEEE International Conference on*, pages 476–483. IEEE, 2015.

135. Kirill Degtyarenko, Paula De Matos, Marcus Ennis, Janna Hastings, Martin Zbinden, Alan McNaught, Rafael Alcántara, Michael Darsow, Mickaël Guedj, and Michael Ashburner. Chebi: a database and ontology for chemical entities of biological interest. *Nucleic acids research*, 36(suppl_1):D344–D350, 2007.

136. The Gene Ontology Consortium. Go-ontology tracking system. https://github.com/geneontology/go-ontology/issues, 2022. [Online; Accessed 23 Jan 2022].

137. Moyra Lawrence, Sylvain Daujat, and Robert Schneider. Lateral thinking: how histone modifications regulate gene expression. *Trends in Genetics*, 32(1):42–56, 2016.

138. Jeremy Rogers and Olivier Bodenreider. Snomed ct: Browsing the browsers. In *KR-MED*, pages 30–36, 2008.

139. National Library of Medicine. Nlm snomed ct browser. https://uts.nlm.nih.gov/, 2019. Accessed: 2019-01.

140. Michael Burch and Steffen Lohmann. Visualizing the evolution of ontologies: A dynamic graph perspective. In *VOILA@ ISWC*, page 69, 2015.

141. Guo-Qiang Zhang, Shiqiang Tao, Ningzhou Zeng, and Licong Cui. Ontologies as nested facet systems for human–data interaction. *Semantic Web*, 11(1):79–86, 2020.

142. Licong Cui, Shiqiang Tao, and Guo-Qiang Zhang. A semantic-based approach for exploring consumer health questions using umls. In *AMIA Annual Symposium Proceedings*, volume 2014, page 432. American Medical Informatics Association, 2014.

143. Licong Cui, Rong Xu, Zhihui Luo, Susan Wentz, Kyle Scarberry, and Guo-Qiang Zhang. Multi-topic assignment for exploratory navigation of consumer health information in netwellness using formal concept analysis. *BMC medical informatics and decision making*, 14(1):63, 2014.

144. Licong Cui, Rebecca Carter, and Guo-Qiang Zhang. Evaluation of a novel conjunctive exploratory navigation interface for consumer health information: a crowdsourced comparative study. *Journal of medical Internet research*, 16(2), 2014.

145. Wei Zhu, Shiqiang Tao, Licong Cui, and Guo-Qiang Zhang. Web-based interactive visualization of non-lattice subgraphs (wins) in snomed ct. *AMIA Summits on Translational Science Proceedings*, 2020:740, 2020.

146. Ellen M Voorhees, Donna K Harman, et al. *TREC: Experiment and evaluation in information retrieval*, volume 63. MIT press Cambridge, MA, 2005.

147. P Jonathon Phillips, Harry Wechsler, Jeffery Huang, and Patrick J Rauss. The feret database and evaluation procedure for face-recognition algorithms. *Image and vision computing*, 16(5):295–306, 1998.

148. Brian Alan Johnson, Ryutaro Tateishi, and Nguyen Thanh Hoan. A hybrid pansharpening approach and multiscale object-based image analysis for mapping diseased pine and oak trees. *International journal of remote sensing*, 34(20):6969–6982, 2013.

149. Guo-Qiang Zhang, Yan Huang, and Licong Cui. Can snomed ct changes be used as a surrogate standard for evaluating the performance of its auditing methods? In *AMIA Annual Symposium Proceedings*, volume 2017, page 1903. American Medical Informatics Association, 2017.

Printed in the United States
by Baker & Taylor Publisher Services